Contents

Introduction

"What is perhaps most disturbing is the absence of real progress toward restructuring health care systems to address both quality and cost concerns, or toward applying advances in information technology to improve administrative and clinical processes."

Committee on Quality Health Care in America, Institute of Medicine, 2001[1]

Ten years after the Institute of Medicine published the landmark report, *Crossing the Quality Chasm: A New Health System for the 21st Century*, the United States health care system continues to face opportunities and challenges in restructuring the delivery of care to improve quality and address increasing costs. The challenges are exacerbated by the unsustainable portion of the federal budget which national health care expenditures are consuming. In 2010, former Secretary of Defense Robert Gates said, "Health care costs are eating the Defense Department alive."[2] It is essential that innovative new methods of delivering and paying for care be implemented, and expanded upon, in order to reduce health care costs without compromising (indeed while improving) quality of care.

In this regard, the passage of the 2010 Patient Protection and Affordable Care Act (the ACA) was a watershed in United States health policy. In addition to insurance reforms and coverage expansion, the ACA includes provisions designed to reduce health care costs and test, implement, and support delivery system reform. This report will focus on the implementation by the executive branch of the ACA's delivery system reform provisions. It also will demonstrate the importance of the effort to reduce costs and improve quality, and chronicle current best practices.

We begin by examining the growth in spending in the United States health care system. Next, we define five priority areas of delivery system reform, and identify cost saving opportunities in these areas. Third, we highlight models of delivery system reform that are currently in practice across the country, with particular attention to their effect on health care cost and quality. The fourth section details the ACA's delivery system reform provisions and the status of their implementation. The report concludes with an analysis of the Administration's progress and offers recommendations for steps moving forward.

The salient fact underlying this report is that the drivers of unnecessary and excess cost in the U.S. health care system result from systemic causes. Public insurance programs, private insurance coverage, military and veterans' care, even corporate self-insurance, all are seeing dramatic and continuing cost increases. The problem is system-wide, and the solution must be too.

If these issues are not addressed, policymakers will face increasingly unpleasant and difficult threats to the insurance coverage, both private and public, of millions of Americans. Gail Wilensky, who oversaw Medicare and Medicaid under President George H.W. Bush, said, "If we don't redesign what we are doing, we can't just cut unit reimbursement and think we are somehow going to get a better system."[3] The ACA offers solutions that do not cut benefits or increase premiums, but instead reform systems of health care delivery to improve health outcomes and cost efficiency. The key challenge facing the United States is how quickly, thoroughly, and efficiently the reform of our health care delivery system can be implemented.

ENDNOTES

[1] Committee on Quality Health Care in America, Institute of Medicine. (2001). *Crossing the Quality Chasm: A New Health Care System for the 21st Century*. Washington, DC: National Academies Press.

[2] Gates, R. (2010, May 8). Remarks as delivered by Secretary of Defense Robert M. Gates, Abilene, KS. Retrieved from http://www.defense.gov/speeches/speech.aspx?speechid=1467.

[3] Goldstein, A. (2011, April 13). Obama proposes tighter curbs on health-care spending. *The Washington Post*. Retrieved from http://www.washingtonpost.com/national/obama-proposes-tighter-curbs-on-health-care-for-older-americans/2011/04/13/AFDqJOYD_story.html

CHAPTER ONE

The Growth of Health Care Spending

"Put simply, our health care problem is our deficit problem. Nothing even comes close. Nothing else."

President Obama, 2009[1]

"If you want to be honest with the fiscal problem and the debt, it really is a health care problem."

Congressman Paul Ryan, 2011[2]

One point is clear. While Democrats and Republicans may disagree on the origins of the national debt and deficit, there is broad bipartisan agreement that the key driver of its growth is health care.

Spending on health care in the United States has grown faster than gross domestic product (GDP), inflation, and population for most of the last four decades. The share of GDP devoted to health care has risen steadily from 5.2 percent in 1960 to 17.6 percent in 2009 (Figure 1).[3]

FIGURE 1.

Health Care Spending as a Percentage of Gross

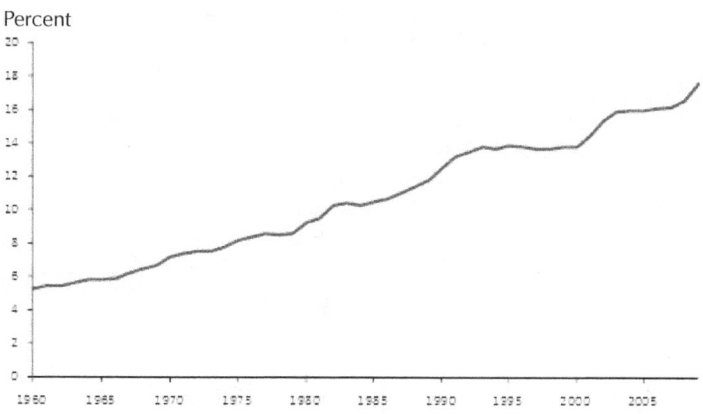

Domestic Product, 1960 to 2009
Source: Centers for Medicare & Medicaid Services. (2009). *National Health Expenditure Data.*

Figure 2 depicts the growth in national health expenditures over the same time period as Figure 1. The growth in health care expenditures puts at risk the long-term fiscal sustainability of the health care system. Health care spending is already limiting the ability of the federal government to invest in other national priorities, such as education, infrastructure, and a clean-energy economy.

FIGURE 2.

National Health Expenditures, 1960 to 2009

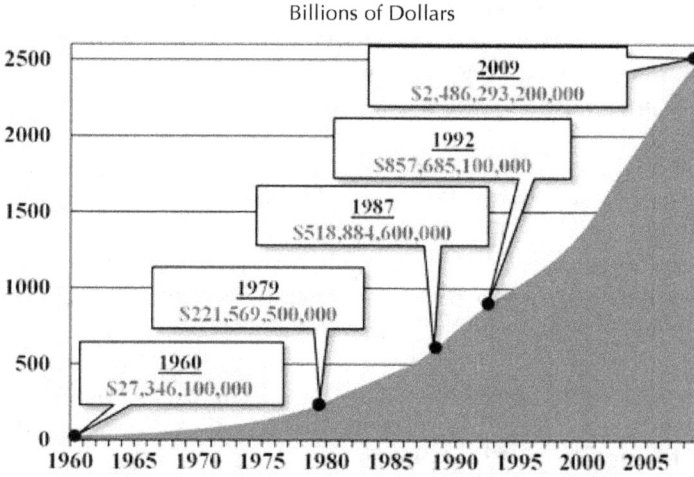

Source: Centers for Medicare & Medicaid Services. (2009). *National Health Expenditure Data.*

In the federal sector, spending on Medicare, Medicaid, the Children's Health Insurance Program, and health insurance subsidies is projected to increase from 5.5 percent of GDP now to almost 14 percent in 2060.[4] If this occurs, the budgetary pressure caused by health care costs will further limit policymakers' options and force painful decisions about limiting benefits or shifting costs to families, states, and the private sector. While limiting benefits or shifting costs may reduce the federal government's health care spending in the short term, these actions fail to provide a sustainable solution to the system-wide health care cost problem. Moreover, these policies have serious implications for businesses and the U.S. economy, individuals' access to care, and the long-term sustainability of the health care system.

In the private sector, rising health care costs have translated into significant premium increases, unemployment, and stagnant real wages. Since 2000, real hourly wage growth net of health benefits has stagnated while inflation-adjusted family health insurance premiums have increased 58 percent.[5] From 2010 to 2011, average annual premiums for employer-sponsored health insurance increased eight percent for single coverage and nine percent for family coverage, costing an average of $5,429 and $15,073 respectively.[6] With the cost of health insurance increasing at this rate, employers and American families are quickly being priced out of coverage. Rising health care costs have also led to reductions in private health insurance coverage, relatively healthy individuals tending to remain uninsured, and erosion of risk-pooling in health insurance markets.[7]

The burden of health care costs on the private sector translates not only into lower wages, but also into less-competitive export products. U.S. automobile manufacturers have testified that health care costs put them at a cost disadvantage relative to Japanese car makers on the order of $1,000 to $1,500 per car.[8, 9]

The rise in health care costs can be in part attributed to the development and adoption of new medical treatments, rising personal income, population aging, and other demographic factors. **However, overpriced and unnecessary services, inefficiently delivered care, excessive administrative costs, missed prevention opportunities, and medical fraud all contribute excessive health care costs that could be reduced without harming – indeed likely improving – the quality of care that Americans receive.[10]**

Health Care Cost Growth by Category of Service

The increase in health care cost varies substantially by category of health service (Figure 3). From 1960 to 2005, national expenditures on hospital services and professional services (i.e. physician services, nurse services, etc.) experienced steep increases. According to the Congressional Budget Office (CBO), hospital and professional services account for most of the long-term growth in total health care spending.[11] Furthermore, CBO notes that when spending growth has slowed (i.e. the mid-1990s) it has primarily been a function of slower growth in these categories.[12]

FIGURE 3.

National Health Expenditures by Service Type, 1960 to 2009

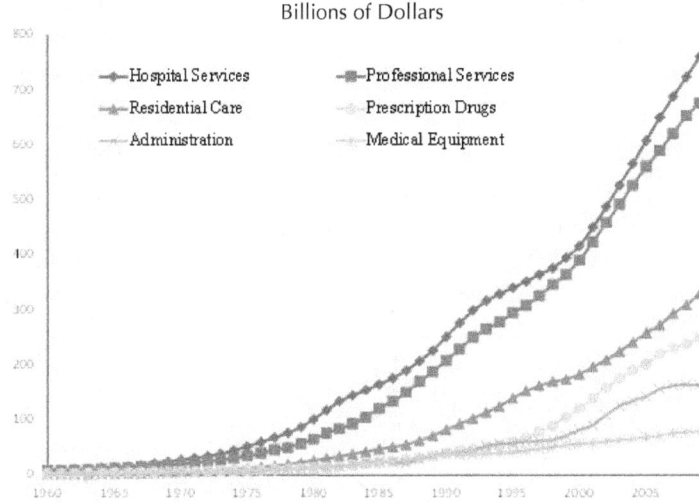

Source: Centers for Medicare & Medicaid Services. (2009). *National Health Expenditure Data.*

Notes: The "Professional Services" series includes "Physician and Clinical," "Dental Services," and "Other Professional Services" categories from the National Health Expenditure Accounts. The "Residential Care" series includes "Home Health Care," "Nursing Care Facilities and Continuing Care Retirement Communities," and "Other Health, Residential and Personal Care." The "Medical Equipment" series includes "Non-Durable Medical Products" and "Durable Medical Equipment." In addition to these categories, this chart excludes data on "Public Health Activity" and "Investment." Expenditures are not adjusted for inflation.

Several provisions of the ACA target the hospital and physician delivery system to promote higher-quality care and restrain health care cost growth. By changing practice and payment patterns, these types of delivery system reforms have the potential to drive value, encourage innovation, and improve efficiency and effectiveness across the entire health care system.

It should also be noted that in 2009, one percent of the population accounted for 21.8 percent of health spending; an average cost of over $90,000 per person.[13] The same report found that five percent of the population accounted for nearly 50 percent of the national health care costs.[14] This suggests that a focus on preventing chronic disease and improving the care of high-utilization patients, such as those with multiple and/or chronic conditions, can yield disproportionate savings in overall system cost.

Variation in Health Care Across the U.S.

Further evidence of delivery system dysfunction is evidenced by the variation in utilization, quality, and spending within the United States. Researchers at Dartmouth University use Medicare data to highlight variation in health care, its causes, and consequences at the state and local levels.[15] Their most recent data, presented in the *Dartmouth Atlas of Health Care*, show that Medicare spending per beneficiary (after adjustment for geographic pricing differences) varies more than twofold between the highest and lowest spending regions. Similar patterns in the utilization rates of specific categories such as surgical procedures, hospitalizations, and primary care visits are apparent. The existence of such wide variation (which persists after accounting for differences in population characteristics) suggests overuse of health care services in some areas.

This conclusion is supported by analyses of the association between spending and quality of care. Figure 4 is reproduced from a 2004 *Health Affairs* article that examined the correlation between quality and Medicare spending with a focus on the role of workforce issues.[16] The chart shows a negative relationship between the quality of care in a state and the level of Medicare spending. That is, higher spending was associated with lower quality. The authors conclude, "The negative relationship between spending and quality and the factors that drive it are of immediate concern." The variation between cost and quality measures suggests that significant improvements in care delivery are possible. Properly-aligned incentives are needed to motivate health care organizations in states that fall in the bottom right of the quality-spending graph in Figure 4 to deliver health care like those in the top left.

While the data analyzed by Baicker and Chandra are now ten years old, the underlying patterns persist in updated analyses of geographic variation conducted by the *Dartmouth Atlas of Health Care*.

International Comparisons of Health Care Spending

The United States is a clear outlier when it comes to health care spending per capita. As seen in Figure 5, data from the Organization for Economic Cooperation and Development (OECD) show that the United States spent $7,960 per capita on health care in 2009, approximately 50 percent higher than the next costliest OECD country, Norway. When compared to neighboring Canada, the United States spent 82 percent more per capita.

FIGURE 5.

Per Capita Health Care Expenditures, 2009 (US$ Purchasing Power Parity)

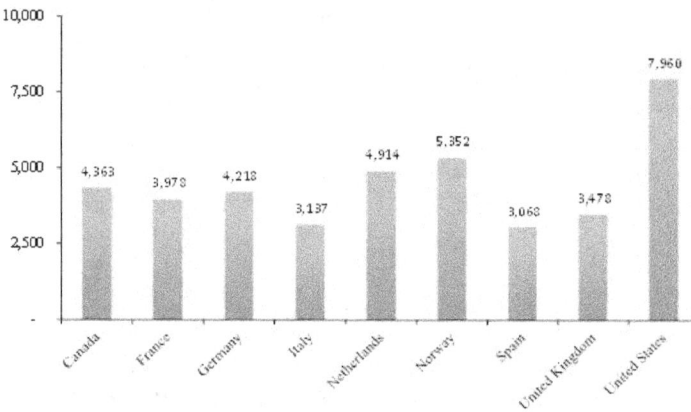

Source: Organization for Economic Cooperation and Development. (2011). Health Expenditure and Financing Data.

Notes: OECD data available at http://stats.oecd.org/index. aspx?DataSetCode=HEALTH_STAT.

Although the United States continues to overspend on health care compared to its peer countries, international studies of health care quality suggest that the United States health care system is underperforming. An analysis by the Commonwealth Fund compared the United States with Australia, Canada, Germany, New Zealand, and the United Kingdom, and ranked our health care system last or next-to-last on five dimensions: quality, access, efficiency, equity, and healthy lives.[17]

The high cost and poor performance of the U.S. health care system raises red flags about the value of our health care spending. On the positive side, however, it suggests that the health care delivery system can yield significant savings and improve health outcomes. **As we discuss further in following chapters, responsible savings estimates range between $700 billion[18] and $1 trillion per year.[19]**

ENDNOTES

1 Obama, B. (2009, September 9). *Remarks by the President to a joint session of Congress on health care.* Speech presented at the U.S. Capitol, Washington, DC. Retrieved from http://www.whitehouse.gov/the_press_office/Remarks-by-the-President-to-a-Joint-Session-of-Congress-on-Health-Care

2 Taylor, A. (2011, March 10). Health care benefit cuts being mapped out by House Republicans. *Huffington Post.* Retrieved from http://www.huffingtonpost.com/2011/03/10/health-care-benefit-cuts-_n_834335.html

3 Centers for Medicare & Medicaid Services. (2009). *National Health Expenditure Data.* Retrieved from https://www.cms.gov/NationalHealthExpendData/downloads/tables.pdf

4 Baicker, K., & Skinner, J. (2011). Health care spending growth and the future of U.S. tax rates. *Tax Policy and the Economy,* 25(1).

5 Baicker, K., & Chandra, A. (2006). The labor market effects of rising health insurance premiums. *Journal of Labor Economics,* 24(3), 609-634.

6 The Kaiser Family Foundation and the Health Research & Educational Trust. (2011, September). *Employer health benefits 2011 annual survey.* Retrieved from http://ehbs.kff.org/pdf/2011/8225.pdf

7 Gilmer T., & Kronick, R. (2005). It's the premiums, stupid: Projections of the uninsured through 2013. *Health Affairs, W5,* 143-151.

8 Daimler Chrysler. (2006, June 6). Statement by Tom LaSorda, President and CEO, Chrysler Group [Press Release], Retrieved from http://cgcomm.daimlerchrysler.com/documents.do?method=display&docType=pressrelease&docId=6946

9 Cooney, S & Yacobucci, B. (2007). *U.S. automotive industry: Policy overview and recent history.* New York: Novinka Books.

10 Institute of Medicine. (2010). The health care imperative: *Lowering costs and improving outcomes: Workshop series summary.* Washington, DC: National Academies Press. Retrieved from http://www.nap.edu/openbook.php?record_id=12750&page=1

11 Congressional Budget Office. (2008, January). *Technological change and the growth of health care spending.* (No. 2764). Retrieved from http://www.cbo.gov/sites/default/files/cbofiles/ftpdocs/89xx/doc8947/01-31-techhealth.pdf

12 Ibid.

13 Cohen, S. & Yu, W. (2012). *The concentration and persistence in the level of health expenditures over time: Estimates for the U.S. population, 2007-2008.* Agency for Healthcare Research and Quality, Statistical Brief No. 354. Retrieved from http://meps.ahrq.gov/mepsweb/data_files/publications/st354/stat354.pdf

14 Cohen, S. &Yu, W. (2012, January). *The concentration and persistence in the level of health expenditures over time: Estimates for the U.S. population, 2007-2008.* Agency for Healthcare Research and Quality, Statistical Brief No. 354. Retrieved from http://meps.ahrq.gov/mepsweb/data_files/publications/st354/stat354.pdf

15 See http://www.dartmouthatlas.org for information on this line of research, and a bibliography of published papers and reports.

16 Baicker, K., & Chandra, A. (2004). Medicare spending, the physician workforce, and beneficiaries' quality of care. *Health Affairs, W4,* 184-197.

17 Davis, K., Schoen, C., Schoenbaum, S., Doty, M., Holmgren, A., Kriss, J., & Shea, K. (2007). *Mirror, mirror on the wall: An international update on the comparative performance of American health care.* New York: The Commonwealth Fund. Retrieved from http://www.commonwealthfund.org/~/media/Files/Publications/Fund%20Report/2007/May/Mirror%20%20Mirror%20on%20the%20Wall%20%20An%20International%20Update%20on%20the%20Comparative%20Performance%20of%20American%20Healt/1027_Davis_mirror_mirror_international_update_v2.pdf

18 Executive Office of the President, Council of Economic Advisers. (2009, June). *The economic case for health care reform.* Retrieved from http://www.whitehouse.gov/administration/eop/cea/TheEconomicCaseforHealthCareReform/

19 O'Neill, P. (2009, July 5). Health care's infectious losses. *New York Times.* Retrieved from http://www.nytimes.com/2009/07/06/opinion/06oneill.html [See also Chapter 2: endnotes 62, 63, and 64].

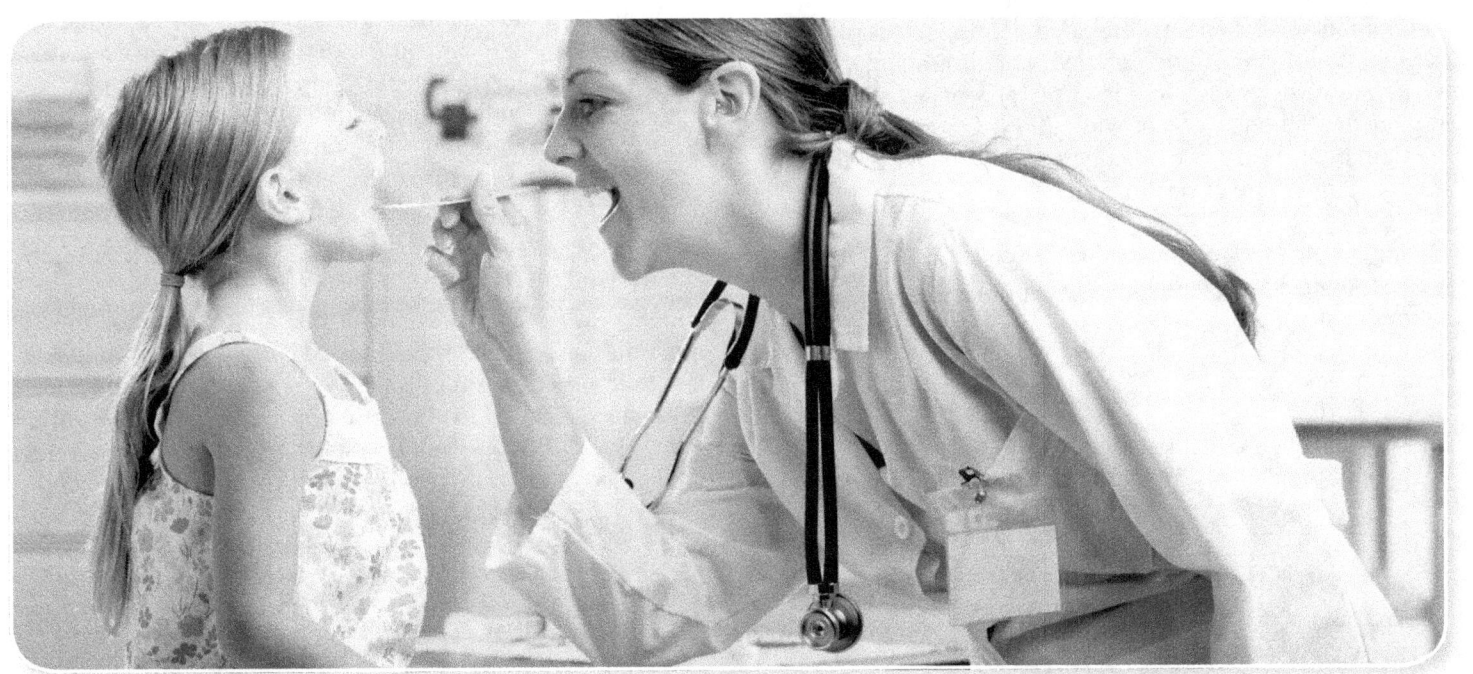

CHAPTER TWO

The Potential of Delivery System Reform

The U.S. health care system has helped Americans live longer and live better since the 1950s. Improvements in medical technology – including new prescription drugs, diagnostics, and treatments – have allowed doctors to treat many illnesses more effectively.[1] However, the health care delivery system remains highly inefficient. According to one estimate, one-third of all spending on health care in the United States may be unnecessary.[2] Reducing one-third of health care spending would bring the U.S. closer to the next least-efficient developed country, Netherlands, which spends 12 percent of its GDP on health care.[3] Identifying and eliminating such vast unnecessary spending should be a high priority.

Much inefficiency can be traced to misaligned incentives, lack of price and quality transparency, and inadequate mechanisms for coordinating and optimizing health care across the continuum of care. **Realigning the delivery system to drive out inefficiencies in the health care system will be key to reducing costs and improving the quality of care.** Five priority areas for delivery system reform commend themselves: (1) payment reform; (2) primary and preventive care; (3) measuring and reporting quality; (4) administrative simplification; and (5) health information technology. This chapter reviews in each priority area relevant research and relevant reforms included in the ACA.

Priority Area I: Payment Reform

Most health care payments in the U.S. are based on volume of service provided. For physicians, individual services are reimbursed based on a schedule of fees; for hospitals, payments are typically set per diem or per discharge. This system rewards volume and intensity of services rather than quality or efficiency, and provides the wrong incentives, particularly for care of medically-complex patients who consume a large share of health care resources.

Paying physicians "fee for service" results in higher utilization of services than capitated or salaried models, but with no systematic improvement in quality.[4] Evidence suggests the primary source of waste in the U.S. health care system is from unnecessary care.[5]

Most experts agree that payment reform is essential to realigning the delivery system to provide higher value care.[6]

Cost savings opportunities associated with such reforms are significant. By one estimate from the RAND Corporation, bundled payment (that is, a fixed payment that covers all services for a specific medical condition) alone could deliver a one-time, five percent reduction in cost.[7] Likewise, researchers at Dartmouth have estimated that global payment – that is, payment based on a global budget (e.g., capitation) – for a population under an Accountable Care Organization (ACO)[i] could slow spending growth by one percentage point per year.[8]

Private insurers have already begun piloting and adopting ACO-type, integrated health care delivery models that align incentives through bundled and global payment reforms. In 2010, Blue Shield of California collaborated with Hill Physicians Medical Group and Catholic Healthcare West, California's largest hospital chain, on an ACO pilot program for Californian Public Employees' Retirement System (CalPERS) members in the Sacramento area. In its first year, the Blue Shield ACO reported impressive results: readmissions were reduced by 15 percent, hospital days were reduced by 15 percent, inpatient stays of 20 or more days were reduced by 50 percent, and total savings amounted to $15.5 million. Part of the savings went toward keeping CalPERS' members premium rates from increasing, and the remainder was shared among the medical providers and Blue Shield.[9]

The Affordable Care Act introduces payment reforms for individual physicians and for larger, organized health care systems, ranging from bundled payments to payment adjustments for hospital-acquired conditions.[ii] Empirical evidence shows that payment structures such as these improve care delivery, costs, and quality. In Chapter 3, we highlight organizations that have successfully implemented payment reforms, and examine the structural and organizational supports that these organizations use to help physicians and other providers to manage population health.

Priority Area II: Primary and Preventive Care

Timely primary and preventive care can improve health outcomes and, in some cases, save money. **Unfortunately, less than one percent of health care spending in the United States goes to clinically-based, effective prevention strategies.**[10] There is evidence suggesting that patients in the United States only receive about half of recommended preventive services.[11] Moreover, the infrastructure for making

---

[i] See the description of the ACO model by Mark McClellan et. al. (2010, May). A national strategy to put accountable care into practice. *Health Affairs*, 29(5), 982-990. "ACOs consist of providers who are jointly held accountable for achieving measured quality improvements and reductions in the rate of spending growth. Our definition emphasizes that these cost and quality improvements must achieve overall, per capita improvements in quality and cost, and that ACOs should have at least limited accountability for achieving these improvements while caring for a defined population of patients."

[ii] See Patient Protection and Affordable Care Act (Pub. L. 111-148) §§ 2702, 2704, 2705, 2706, 2707, 3001, 3006, 3008, 3021, 3022, 3023, 3025, and 3403. (2010).

authoritative determination of the cost and benefit of various preventive strategies is still quite primitive.

For some conditions, compliance with appropriate care is alarmingly low. Individuals with diabetes need glycosylated hemoglobin tests to monitor their condition and reduce preventable hospitalizations; only 24 percent reported receiving three or more of these tests over a two-year period. For individuals suffering from alcohol dependence, rates of compliance were even lower, with only 10.5 percent reporting recommended care.[12]

The failure of patients to receive recommended preventive care can be costly to the U.S. health care system. According to the Centers for Disease Control and Prevention (CDC), when colorectal cancer is found early and treated, the five-year survival rate is 90 percent.[13] Unfortunately, screening rates for colorectal cancer are low: the National Health Interview Survey found that in 2005 only half the population aged 50 and older received recommended screening for colon cancer. The CDC reports that as many as 60 percent of deaths from colorectal cancer could be prevented if everyone age 50 and older were screened regularly.[14] The American Cancer Society has found that increasing colorectal screening rates in the pre-Medicare population could not only save lives, but reduce subsequent Medicare treatment costs by $15 billion over 11 years.[15] Likewise, previous research has shown smoking cessation and influenza vaccination to save lives either at low cost or at a cost savings.[16] Obesity prevention presents another potentially important opportunity. According to a study by the CDC, in 2008, the direct and indirect costs of obesity totaled as much as $147 billion.[17]

In order to shift to a culture of prevention in our health care system, efforts must be made to prioritize and strengthen the primary care system. The primary care infrastructure relied upon to deliver primary and secondary prevention is increasingly strained.[18] **Only six to eight percent of health care spending goes to primary care – less than the percentage that goes to private insurance overhead.**[19] Thus, many patients lack timely access to primary care providers. The income gap between primary care physicians and specialists, coupled with other factors, led to a significant decline in the number of U.S. medical students choosing to pursue careers in primary care.[20]

If these trends continue, access to primary care providers is likely to deteriorate. This is troubling, since for most patients the primary care practitioner is their source of first-contact coverage and their care coordinator.[21] A weak primary care infrastructure is associated with higher hospitalization rates for asthma, diabetes mellitus, chronic obstructive pulmonary disease (COPD), congestive heart failure (CHF), and hypertension;[22] conditions generally best treated most efficiently outside of a hospital setting. Many chronic conditions can be controlled with routine monitoring, counseling, and medication, and hospitalization should only occur in rare cases. Research shows that primary care relieves high emergency department use.[23] Better use of evidence-based preventive care and primary care can result in less need for costly acute care and improved value of health care spending.

The Affordable Care Act includes a number of reforms that realign incentives toward prevention and reinforce the role of primary care providers,[iii] some of which use principles of population health management and enhanced infrastructure such as disease registries and systems for tracking tests and referrals. Several provisions build off of the "medical home" initiative (sometimes called the "patient-centered" or "advanced" medical home), in which primary care practices take greater responsibility for coordinating care for patients across the continuum of specialty and inpatient services.[24]

One example of a patient-centered medical home (PCMH) is the Rhode Island Chronic Care Sustainability Initiative (CSI-RI), one of the country's first statewide, multi-payer, patient-centered medical home pilots.[iv] In addition to improving quality and health outcomes, the CSI-RI pilot was designed to align quality improvement and financial incentives across Rhode Island's health plans, purchasers, and providers, and enhance the attractiveness of entering into primary care.[25] The project started with five primary care sites in 2007 and was expanded to an additional eight primary sites in 2010, reaching a total participation of 79 providers and 70,000 covered lives. CSI-RI is one of eight all-payer, patient-centered medical home projects nationally to be joined by Medicare as a full participating provider through CMS' Multi-payer Advanced Primary Care Program.

A survey taken by staff at pilot sites show that job satisfaction among staff improved from 44 percent to 100 percent between the first and second year of the program.[26] People love it. Moreover, pilot sites, which are required to electronically report clinical quality data as part of their obligations under CSI-RI, have reported the following care improvements over the first four years of the project:

- the percentage of patients with diabetes under control has improved from 32 percent to 66 percent;
- the percentage of patients with coronary artery disease prescribed a beta blocker has improved from 40 percent to 78.7 percent; and
- the percentage of patients screened for depression increased from 7.5 percent to 66.4 percent.[27]

---

iii See Patient Protection and Affordable Care Act (Pub. L. 111-148) §§ 2602, 2703, 3024, 3026, 3146, 3502, 3503, 4001, 4108, 4201, 4202, 5604, and 10333. (2010).

iv Under CSR-RI, participating practices receive a per-member-per-month payment from all participating health plans to cover the costs of implementing and maintaining the medical home. The health plans also support the cost of having a nurse care manager on-site in every practice location.

Provisions included in the ACA that strengthen primary care and prevention include the Community Transformation Grant program (§4201), as well as a program to fund community health teams to support the development of primary care practices into medical homes (§3502). In addition, the Center for Medicare and Medicaid Innovation (CMMI) (§3021) is administering the Comprehensive Primary Care Initiative, a program to strengthen primary care practices and help primary care doctors deliver better-coordinated care. Under this initiative, CMS is working with public and private payers to offer a bonus payment or monthly care-management fee to participating primary care doctors who coordinate care for their Medicare patients. When targeted effectively at high-risk patients and preventable, high-cost events, such efforts can reduce total health care costs while improving quality, as demonstrated in recent evaluations of patient-centered medical homes.[28]

Priority Area III: Measuring and Reporting Quality

U.S. health care data shows that the health care system is riddled with opportunities for quality improvement in areas such as chronic disease management, prevention, safety, efficiency, and patient experience.[29] **Systematically measuring and reporting health care quality is an essential first step.**[30] Accurate and reliable quality information can be a vital resource for providers to improve their own practices, for patients and insurers to make informed decisions, and for delivery system improvement generally. Knowing more about quality differences between providers will encourage healthy and value-based competition.

Without quality information, it is difficult for a consumer to know whether the price of a service reflects real value toward improving his or her health outcomes, or simply the provider's market power. Even though data suggest there is little connection between cost and quality in health care,[31] many consumers today assume that high prices in health care signal better quality. Quality information gives consumers the tools to be better informed about the type of services that best fit their care needs.

Efforts to incentivize high-performance physicians and hospitals by insurers eager to reward high-quality, low-cost care have been hampered by challenges in consistently measuring quality.[32] To improve consistency and address gaps in quality measurement, the Affordable Care Act includes provisions requiring the Secretary of Health and Human Services, the Agency for Healthcare Research and Quality, and the Centers for Medicare & Medicaid Services, among other entities, to identify, update, and expand health quality measures; to publicly report these efforts; and to develop strategic plans for health care quality.[v] In addition, quality measurement and improvement are key components to ACA payment and care coordination reforms such as

the Hospital Value-Based Purchasing Program (§3001); the Medicare Shared Savings Program (§3022); the Value-Base Payment Modifier for Physicians (§3007); and the CMS Innovation Center's Partnership for Patients Initiative (§3021). The integration of quality measurement and quality improvement goals in so many of the ACA's delivery system reforms reflects their importance to improving the delivery of health services and patient outcomes.

Priority Area IV: Administrative Simplification

The proportion of the U.S. health care dollar lost to administration has traditionally been high relative to peer countries.[33] **The cost of administration by insurance companies is high, and the "shadow cost" imposed on providers is probably even higher.** Unfortunately, evidence suggests that this gap is growing. A series of comparisons has revealed that administrative costs in the United States are nearly three times higher than in Canada.[34] According to this research, between 1969 and 1999 the share of the U.S. health care labor force accounted for by administrative workers grew from 18.2 percent to 27.3 percent.[35] This was considerably higher than growth in Canada, where the administrative share of the health care labor force rose from 16.0 percent in 1971 to 19.1 percent in 1996. These figures may be subject to

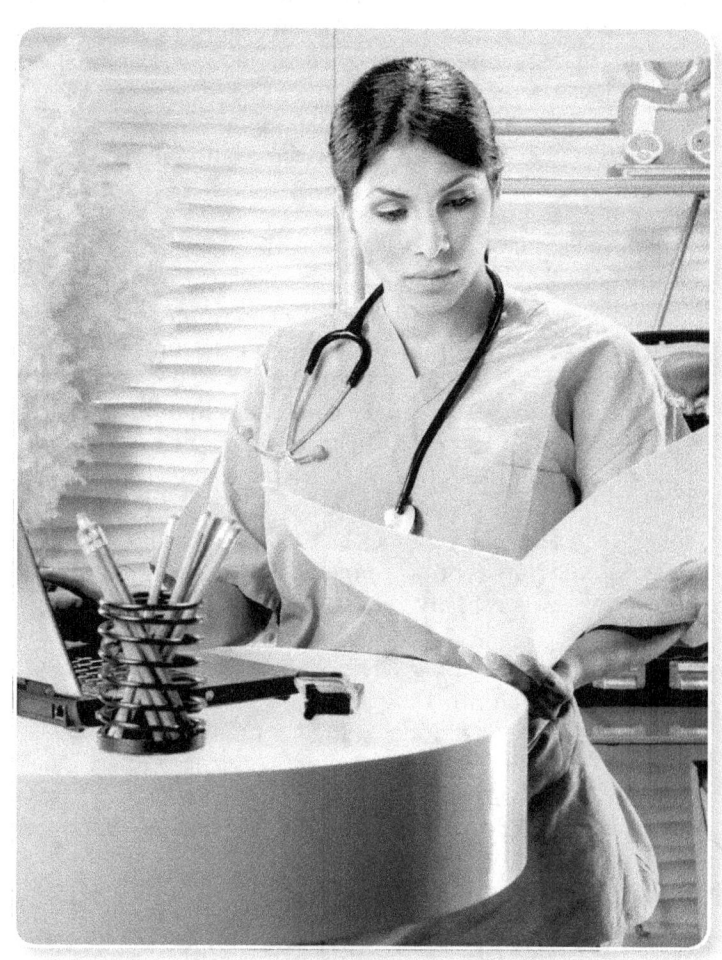

---

v   See Patient Protection and Affordable Care Act (Pub. L. 111-148) §§ 2701, 3004, 3005, 3011, 3012, 3013, 3014, 3015, 6301, and 10322. (2010).

some measurement error,[36] but the differences between the United States and other countries are stark and the burden of administrative costs in the health care system is undeniably growing.

For hospitals, the challenge of operating in a complex health care system with numerous payers, regulations, and patients has necessitated large expenditures on administrative personnel. In 1968, U.S. hospitals employed 435,100 managers and clerks to support the care of 1,378,000 inpatients daily. In 1990, the average number of daily inpatients had fallen to 853,000 and the number of administrative staff had risen to 1,221,600:[37] the administrative staff rose to outnumber the patients. One recent paper reported that for every office-based physician in the U.S. there are 2.2 administrative workers; for every hospital bed there are 1.5 administrative workers.[38] Notably, the U.S. has approximately 25 percent more administrative workers in health care than the U.K. and 215 percent more than Germany, despite having similar numbers of clinical personnel (all on a per capita basis).

Some administrative costs are associated with important quality improvement or cost control efforts. For example, pay-for-performance payment reforms place an additional administrative burden on providers, including the time it takes doctors to properly report quality measures.[39] While not all administrative costs are wasteful, plenty are. For example, the multiplicity and intricacy of health care payment systems in the U.S. has resulted in a proliferation of billing forms and systems for submitting paper and electronic bills. This proliferation creates additional work for providers with little to no added value. Opportunities for savings in this area are significant. A study published in *Health Affairs* documented that physicians spent on average 142 hours annually interacting with health plans, totaling nearly seven percent of total health care costs.[40] And that doesn't count the non-physician office staff.

Easing the administrative burden on health care providers – particularly the back and forth between providers and insurers on approvals and claims reimbursement – can reduce costs and improve efficiency in the health care system. The Affordable Care Act promotes uniform electronic communication between providers and insurers for the purposes of patient eligibility verification, claims status inquires and payment, and referral authorization requests, among other functions.[vi] The law also requires a single, streamlined form to be used in each state that will enable consumers to apply for available State health subsidy programs. These types of reforms will help reduce personnel and time spent resolving administrative paperwork, leading to a more efficient and cost-effective health care system.

Priority Area V: Health Information Technology

Health information technology (IT) will radically transform the health care industry, and is the essential, underlying framework for health care delivery system reform. The ACA's payment reforms, pilot projects, and other delivery system reforms are built with the expectation of having IT-enabled providers. In particular, the shift to new models of care, like ACOs, will rely heavily on information exchange and reporting quality outcomes. Indeed, the formation of ACOs is contingent on having providers "online" to transfer information and patient records, and report quality measures.

As the ACA's delivery system reforms are implemented, providers will look for new ways to engage patients with their health information, to analyze and report data, and connect with other providers. Health IT will enable doctors to update vital information in real time, access the best illness, prevention, and treatment information and strategies, and keep patients better informed and engaged. Health IT is key to coordination of care and essential to enabling new payment systems; all four of the priority areas depend on health IT to succeed.

Health IT can raise quality, improve health outcomes and reduce cost.[41] Health IT allows for better information management, an important step in delivering high-quality care.[42] The adoption of health IT is also associated with improvement in patient safety.[43,44] **In 2000, the Institute of Medicine estimated the number of deaths resulting from medical error as high as 98,000 deaths annually.**[45] The most common causes of preventable injuries (and deaths) in hospitals – medication errors – can be reduced through the adoption of computerized physician order entry (CPOE) systems. The implementation of CPOE systems is associated with a reduction in medication errors of 55 percent.[46,47]

Despite evidence that health IT is effective, widespread adoption of new IT has moved slowly in the United States.[48,49,50,51] In an article published in 2005, John Chambers, CEO of Cisco Systems, said that the health care industry ". . . is down there with mining as the most technophobic industry."[52] In the same article, Jeff Miller, a manager at Hewlett Packard, called health care "one of the slowest-adopting industries."[53]

A 2002 survey revealed that only 9.6 percent of U.S. hospitals had CPOE completely available.[54] We lag many of our international competitors: over 80 percent of general practitioners in Australia, the Netherlands, New Zealand, the United Kingdom and Germany have adopted electronic health records, only ten to 30 percent of ambulatory care physicians in the United States use electronic health records.[55]

[vi] See Patient Protection and Affordable Care Act (Pub. L. 111-148) §§ 1104, 1413, and 6105. (2010).

However, these trends are changing thanks to the Health Information Technology for Economic and Clinical Health (HITECH) Act, which was signed into law in 2009 as part of the American Recovery and Reinvestment Act. The HITECH Act took important steps to restructure financial incentives to shift the pattern of health IT adoption. The HITECH Act's Medicare and Medicaid incentive payments are encouraging doctors and hospitals to adopt and "meaningfully use" certified electronic health records.

In February 2012, CMS announced new data which details that the agency has made $3.12 billion in incentive payments to 41,000 physicians, 2,000 hospitals, and other health care providers for the meaningful use of certified EHRs.[56] In the longer term, the Congressional Budget Office (CBO) estimates that these incentives will increase adoption rates to about 70 percent for hospitals and 90 percent for physicians by 2019.[57]

In addition, the HITECH Act established the Health IT Extension Program, which funded regional extension centers to offer technical assistance to accelerate health care providers' efforts and the Beacon Communities Program, which rewards "beacon" communities at the frontier of adopting health IT and health information exchange.[vii] The CBO expects health IT savings to federal programs of approximately $7 billion during the five-year period 2010-2014.[58] The same report suggests that providers will enjoy $17 billion in savings due to efficiency gains in their operations.

The Affordable Care Act includes several provisions directly related to health IT.[viii] Importantly, the ACA includes provisions that advance the HITECH Act's goal of "meaningful use" of electronic health records by incorporating more sophisticated uses of health IT as a central component or requirement. These include the Hospital Value-Based Purchasing Program (§3001(a)), the Medicare Shared Savings Program (§3022), the Medicaid Health Home Option (§2703), and the quality reporting provisions for long-term care facilities, cancer hospitals, and psychiatric hospitals (§3004; §3005; §103022), among others.

As health data is collected and shared across providers, the health care system will move toward a "learning health system."[59] Anonymized patient and claims data can be analyzed for associations and anomalies which otherwise may not be apparent. Awareness of these patterns will help providers understand health care outcomes across populations, target fraud and abuse, and identify variation in care. With an IT-enabled health system, data flow and analysis can occur in "real time," creating a rapid flow of new information on how to achieve what HHS calls the "Triple Aim" – better health, better care, and lower costs.

Finally, a robust health IT infrastructure will allow entrepreneurial development of "apps" to facilitate best-quality care, tailored to personal medical needs, with decision support for providers, and compliance support and transparency for patients (and their caregiver loved ones). Both the "learning health system" and the entrepreneurial development of health care "apps" provide opportunities for emerging industries akin to those that emerged around the Internet, fueling a potential health management technology boom.

Conclusion

There is tremendous potential for improved care and cost savings from the five priority areas of health care delivery system reform: payment reform, primary and preventive care, measuring and reporting quality, administrative simplification, and health information technology. These areas are not separate silos; progress in each area will influence, and be influenced by, progress in others. Innovation in these areas can drive "virtuous cycles" of improvement in care, efficiency in delivery, transparency in information, and reduction in cost. **Various studies that have looked at the collective potential for health care savings from such strategies have arrived at annual savings as high as $700 billion[60]; $765 billion[61]; $850 billion[62]; or even $1 trillion.[63,64]** The following chapter will show how exemplar models of delivery system reform across the country are already affecting health care outcomes and cost trends.

ENDNOTES

[1] Cutler D., & McClellan, M. (2001). Is technological change in medicine worth it? *Health Affairs*, 20, 11-29.

[2] Brownlee, S. (2007). *Overtreated: Why too much medicine is making us sicker and poorer.* New York: Bloomsbury.

[vii] The Rhode Island Quality Institute (RIQI) is the only organization in the nation to win all three of the major ARRA health IT awards from the HITECH Act: the Regional Extension Center program, the Beacon Community program, and the Health Information Exchange program. RIQI's RI Beacon Community Program, a public-private collaboration that aims to improve specific clinical metrics by electronically enabling the Patient-Centered Medical Home (PCMH) and build a statewide quality reporting and analytics capability. Twenty-eight PCMHs met the criteria to participate in the Beacon program, which focuses on reducing preventable hospital use, improving the quality of care for patients with diabetes, reducing tobacco use, and building a robust, statewide data and analytics infrastructure. The Beacon Program enhances the State's ongoing delivery system reform efforts, such as the all-payer PCMH program, by providing practices with health IT tools, such as linkages to the statewide health information exchanges, and services, such as real-time provider notification of the admission or discharge of their patients to a Rhode Island ED or hospital. RIQI operates the RI Regional Extension Center, which is assisting nearly 900 RI providers to achieve the Meaningful Use targets. The RI Regional Extension Center has expanded its services to assisting providers in adopting other innovations that support transformation. RIQI also operates *currentcare*, which enables providers to access and share patients' health information. The system began sharing data in 2010. By the end of this year the system is expected to have 100 percent of the hospitals in the State connected, and contain 90 percent of all prescription data and 88 percent of all laboratory results. Thirty-five percent of Rhode Island's population has voluntarily enrolled in *currentcare* and RIQI has over 400 hospitals, physician offices, long-term care facilities, mental health centers, and visiting nurse agencies as enrollment partners.

[viii] See Patient Protection and Affordable Care Act (Pub. L. 111-148) §§ 1561, 6114, and 10330. (2010).

[3] Organization for Economic Cooperation and Development. (2011). Retrieved from http://www.oecd-ilibrary.org/social-issues-migration-health/total-expenditure-on-health_20758480-table1

[4] Rosenthal, M. (2000). Risk sharing and the supply of mental health services. *Journal of Health Economics, 19*(6), 1047-1065; and Hellinger, F. (1998). The effect of managed care on quality: A review of recent evidence. *Archives of Internal Medicine, 158*(8), 833-841.; and Robinson, J. (2001). Theory and practice in the design of physician payment incentives. *Milbank Quarterly, 79*(2), 149-177.

[5] Brownlee, S. (2007). *Overtreated: Why too much medicine is making us sicker and poorer*. New York: Bloomsbury.

[6] See for example: Cutler, D. (2006, October). Follow the money: Payment reform as the key to health reform. (AARP Public Policy Institute Paper #2006-24). Washington, D.C.: AARP.

[7] Hussey P., Eibner, C., Ridgely, M., & McGlynn, E. (2009). Controlling U.S. health care spending: Separating promising from unpromising approaches. *New England Journal of Medicine, 361*(22), 2109–2111.

[8] Fisher, E., McClellan, M., Bertko, J., Lieberman, S., Lee, J., Lewis, J., & Skinner, J. (2009). Fostering accountable health care: Moving forward in Medicare. *Health Affairs, 28*(2), w219–w231.

[9] Blue Shield of California. "Fact Sheet: Blue Shield of California and Accountable Care Organizations (ACOs)." Retrieved from https://www.blueshieldca.com/bsca/documents/about-blue-shield/health-reform/ACO_Blue_Shield_Fact_Sheet_72811.pdf

[10] Partnership to Fight Chronic Disease. (2009). *Almanac of Chronic Disease*. Retrieved from http://www.fightchronicdisease.org/sites/default/files/docs/2009AlmanacofChronicDisease_updated81009.pdf

[11] McGlynn, E., Asch, S., Adams, J., Keesey, J., Hicks, J., DeCristofaro, A., & Kerr, E. (2003). The quality of health care delivered to adults in the United States. *New England Journal of Medicine, 348*, 2635–2645.

[12] Ibid.

[13] Centers for Disease Control and Prevention. *Colorectal cancer screening rates*. Retrieved from http://www.cdc.gov/cancer/colorectal/statistics/screening_rates.htm

[14] Ibid.

[15] National Colorectal Cancer Roundtable. (2007, September). *Increasing colorectal cancer screening – Saving lives and saving dollars: Screening 50 to 64 year olds reduces cancer costs to Medicare*. Retrieved from http://action.acscan.org/site/DocServer/Increasing_Colorectal_Cancer_Screening_-_Saving_Lives_an.pdf?docID=18927

[16] Maciosek, M., Coffield, A., Edwards, N., Flottemesch, T., Goodman, M., & Solberg, L. (2006). Priorities among effective clinical preventive services: Results of a systematic review and analysis. *American Journal of Preventative Medicine, 31*, 52-61.

[17] Centers for Disease Control. (2011). Obesity – Halting the epidemic: At a glance. Retrieved from http://www.cdc.gov/chronicdisease/resources/publications/aag/obesity.htm

[18] Bodenheimer, T. (2006). Primary care: Will it survive? *New England Journal of Medicine, 355*, 861-864.

[19] Goroll, A., Berenson, R.,Schoenbaum, S., and Gardner, L. (2007, January). Fundamental reform of payment for adult primary care: Comprehensive payment for comprehensive care. *Journal of General Internal Medicine*.

[20] American College of Physicians (2006, January 30). *The impending collapse of primary care medicine and its implications for the state of the nation's health care*. Retrieved from http://www.acponline.org/advocacy/events/state_of_healthcare/statehc06_1.pdf

[21] Grumbach, K. (1999). Resolving the gatekeeper conundrum. *Journal of the American Medical Association, 282*(3), 261-266.

[22] Oster, A., & Bindman, A. (2003). Emergency department visits for ambulatory care sensitive conditions: Insights into preventable hospitalizations. *Medical Care, 41*(2), 198–207; and Falik, M., Needleman, J., Wells, B., &

Korb, J. (2001). Ambulatory care sensitive hospitalizations and emergency visits: Experiences of Medicaid patients using federally qualified health centers. *Medical Care, 39*(6), 551-561.

[23] Ibid; Grumbach, K., Keane, D., & Bindman, A. (1993). Primary care and public emergency department overcrowding. *American Journal of Public Health, 83*(3), 372-378.

[24] American Academy of Family Physicians, American College of Physicians, American Osteopathic Association, American Academy of Pediatrics. (2007, February). *Joint principles of the patient-centered medical home*. Retrieved from http://www.pcpcc.net/content/joint-principles-patient-centered-medical-home

[25] Office of the Health Insurance Commissioner. (2010). *The Rhode Island Chronic Care Sustainability Initiative: A multi-payer demonstration of the patient-centered medical home*. Retrieved from http://www.ohic.ri.gov/documents/Committees/CSI%202011/Snapshot%20of%20CSI%20%20-%20Jan%202011.pdf

[26] Rosenthal, M. (2011). Presentation of preliminary findings of evaluation of CSI-RI.

[27] Ibid.

[28] Reid, R., Coleman, K., Johnson, E., Fishman, P., Hsu, C., Soman, M., . . . Larson, E. (2010). The group health medical home at year two: cost savings, higher patient satisfaction, and less burnout for providers. *Health Affairs, 29*(5), 835 – 843.

[29] Institute of Medicine. (2001). *Crossing the quality chasm: A new health system for the twenty-first century*. Washington, D.C.: National Academy Press.

[30] Donabedian, A. (1988). The quality of care: How can it be assessed? *Journal of the American Medical Association, 260*(12), 1743–1748.

[31] Baicker, K., & Chandra, A. (2004). Medicare spending, the physician workforce, and beneficiaries' quality of care. *Health Affairs, W4*, 184–197.

[32] Epstein, A. (1998). Rolling down the runway: The challenges ahead for quality report cards. *Journal of the American Medical Association, 279*(21), 1691-1696.

[33] Woolhandler, S., & Himmelstein, D. (1991). The deteriorating administrative efficiency of the U.S. health care system. *New England Journal of Medicine, 324*, 1253-1258.

[34] Ibid; Woolhandler,S., Campbell, T., & Himmelstein, D. (2003). Costs of health care administration in the United States and Canada. *New England Journal of Medicine, 349*, 768-775.

[35] Ibid.

[36] Aaron, H. (2003). The cost of health care administration in the United States and Canada: Questionable answers to a questionable question. *New England Journal of Medicine, 349*, 801-803.

[37] Woolhandler, S., Himmelstein, D., & Lewontin, J. (1993). Administrative costs in U.S. hospitals. *New England Journal of Medicine, 329*, 400-403.

[38] Cutler, D., & Ly D. (2011). The (paper)work of medicine: Understanding international medical costs. *Journal of Economic Perspectives, 25*(2), 3-25.

[39] Morra, D., Nicholson, S., Levinson, W., Gans, D., Hammons, T., & Casalino L. (2011). US physician practices versus Canadians: Spending nearly four times as much money interacting with payers. *Health Affairs, 30*(8), 1443-1450.

[40] Casalino, L., Nicholson, S., Gans, D., Hammons, T., Morra, D., Karrison, T., & Levinson, W. (2009). What does it cost physician practices to interact with health insurance plans? *Health Affairs, 28*(4), w533-w543.

[41] Goldzweig, C., Towfigh, A., Maglione, M., & Shekelle, P. (2009). Costs and benefits of health information technology: New trends from the literature. *Health Affairs, 28*(2), w282-w293.

[42] Chassin, M., Galvin RW. (1998). The urgent need to improve health care quality: Institute of Medicine National Roundtable on Health Care Quality. *Journal of the American Medical Association, 280*(11), 1000-1005.

[43] Bates, D., Leape, L., Cullen, D., Laird, N., Petersen, L., Teich, J., . . . Seger, D. (1998). Effect of computerized physician order entry and a team intervention on prevention of serious medication errors. *Journal of the American Medical Association, 280*(15), 1311-1316.

[44] Bates, D., & Gawande, A. (2003). Improving safety with information technology. *New England Journal of Medicine, 348*, 2526-2534.

[45] Kohn, L., Corrigan, J., & Donaldson, M. (Eds.). (1999). *To err is human: Building a safer health system.* Washington, DC: National Academy Press.

[46] Bates, D., Leape, L., Cullen, D., Laird, N., Petersen, L., Teich, J., . . . Seger, D. (1998). Effect of computerized physician order entry and a team intervention on prevention of serious medication errors. *Journal of the American Medical Association, 280*(15), 1311-1316.

[47] Teich, J., Glaser, J., Beckley, R., Aranow, M., Bates, D., Kuperman, G., . . . Spurr, C. (1996). Toward cost-effective, quality care; the Brigham Integrated Computing System. Retrieved from http://www.himss.org/content/files/davies_1996_brigham.pdf.

[48] DesRoches, C., Campbell, E., Rao, S., Donelan, K., Ferris, T., Jha, A., . . . Blumenthal, D. (2008). Electronic health records in ambulatory care: A national survey of physicians. *New England Journal of Medicine, 359*, 50-60.

[49] Jha, A., DesRoches, C., Campbell, E., Donelan, K., Rao, S., Ferris, T., . . . Blumenthal, D. (2009). Use of electronic health records in U.S. hospitals. *New England Journal of Medicine, 360*, 1628-1638.

[50] Institute of Medicine. (2001). Crossing the quality chasm: A new health system for the 21st century. Washington, DC: National Academy Press.

[51] Ash, J., Gorman, P., Seshadri, V., & Hersh, W. (2004). Computerized physician order entry in U.S. hospitals: Results of a 2002 survey. *Journal of the American Medical Informatics Association, 11*, 95-99.

[52] *Economist.* (2005, April 28). The no-computer virus. Retrieved from http://www.economist.com/node/3909439.

[53] Ibid.

[54] Ash, J., Gorman, P., Seshadri, V., & Hersh, W. (2004). Computerized physician order entry in U.S. hospitals: Results of a 2002 survey. *Journal of the American Medical Informatics Association, 11*, 95-99.

[55] Jha, A., Doolan, D., Grandt, D., Scott, T., & Bates, D. (2008). The use of health information technology in seven nations. *International Journal of Medical Informatics, 77*(12), 848-854.

[56] Centers for Medicare & Medicaid Services. (2012, January). *EHR Incentive Program: Active registrations.* Retrieved from http://www.cms.gov/EHRIncentivePrograms/Downloads/Monthly_Payment_Registration_Report_Updated.pdf

[57] Redhead, S. (2009, April 27). *The Health Information Technology for Economic and Clinical Hope Act.* Congressional Research Service.

[58] Congressional Budget Office. (2008, December). *Budget options, Volume I: Health care.* Retrieved from http://www.cbo.gov/ftpdocs/99xx/doc9925/12-18-HealthOptions.pdf

[59] Office of the National Coordinator for Health Information Technology. *Federal health information technology strategic plan, 2011-2015.* Retrieved from http://healthit.hhs.gov/portal/server.pt/gateway/PTARGS_0_0_4318_1211_15583_43/http%3B/wci-pubcontent/publish/onc/public_communities/f_j/onc_website___home/fed_health_strategic_plan/fed_health_it_strategic_plan_home_portlet/files/final_federal_health_it_strategic_plan_0911.pdf

[60] Executive Office of the President, Council of Economic Advisers. (2009, June). *The economic case for health care reform.* Retrieved from http://www.whitehouse.gov/assets/documents/CEA_Health_Care_Report.pdf

[61] Institute of Medicine. (2011, February 24). The healthcare imperative: Lowering costs and improving outcomes – Workshop series summary. Washington, DC: National Academies Press.

[62] Delaune, J., & Everett, W. (2008). *Waste and inefficiency in the U.S. health care system.* Cambridge, MA: New England Healthcare Institute.

[63] Simon, C., Wolcott, J., & Hogan, P. (2009, October 26). Can we reduce health care spending? Searching for low-hanging fruit in the garden of health system reform. The Lewin Group. Retrieved from http://www.ingenix.com/~/media/Ingenix/Resources/Articles/LewinReportCostDrivers.pdf

[64] O'Neill, P. (2009, July 5). Health care's infectious losses. *New York Times.* Retrieved from http://www.nytimes.com/2009/07/06/opinion/06oneill.html

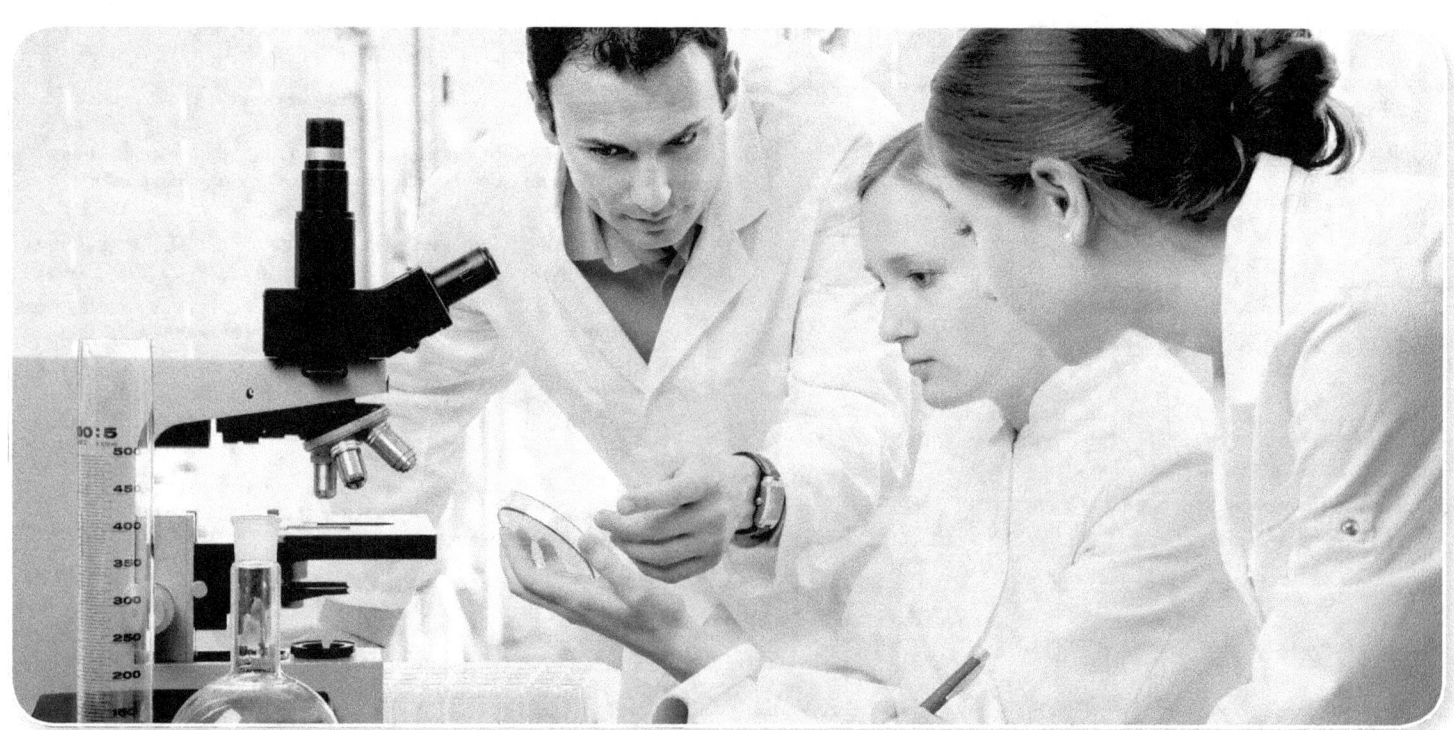

CHAPTER THREE

Delivery System Reform Exemplars

The previous chapter reviewed the five priority areas for delivery system reform: payment reform, primary and preventive care, measuring and reporting quality, administrative simplification, and health information technology. The next chapter will review how the Affordable Care Act authorizes a number of delivery system reforms that are crucial to improving the sustainability of the health care system. However, innovation and reform of care delivery models are not limited to the federal government. This chapter describes real-world examples of initiatives in each of these key areas.

The exemplars include programs implemented by Geisinger Health System in Pennsylvania, Vermont Blueprint for Health, Intermountain Healthcare in Utah and Idaho, and the Marshfield Clinic in Wisconsin. Each of these initiatives is part of a growing national movement of providers, payers, and states dedicated to improving the quality, safety, and effectiveness of care; pioneering new delivery systems that encourage providers to better coordinate care; and reducing waste and inefficiency.

While this chapter highlights each exemplar through the lens of one of the five priority areas, it is important to note that the success each program has achieved is the result of system-wide improvement efforts that span other priority areas. The priority areas we define are not meant to stand alone. Rather, as noted in Chapter 2, progress in each priority area will influence, and be influenced by, progress in other areas in a manner that can drive "virtuous cycles" of improvement in care, efficiency in delivery, transparency in information, and reduction in cost.

From the real-life examples in this chapter, we can draw lessons for the implementation of delivery system reform across the entire health care system; these reforms have worked in improving the quality and reducing the cost of care.

Priority Area I: Payment Reform

Innovation through payment reform is essential to curb spending and to improve the incentives to deliver appropriate, safe, and effective care. Geisinger Health System provides a model for success in reducing costs by marrying payment reforms to care delivery.

Geisinger Health System Background

Geisinger Health System (Geisinger) is a physician-led, integrated delivery system located in central and northeastern Pennsylvania. It employs over 1,000 physicians across 55 practice sites and owns five acute care hospitals and other specialty facilities. The system serves approximately 2.6 million residents from 43 counties who, on average, are poorer, sicker, and older than the rest of the national population.[1] Geisinger also owns and operates its own health maintenance organization, Geisinger Health Plan, consisting of 295,000 members. (The author notes an apparent correlation between health systems that are on both sides of the payer-provider divide and those that are most forward on system reform.)

Payment Reform: Geisinger's Exploration of Two Models

In 2004, Geisinger developed a unique brand of provider reimbursement, building off of a pay-for-performance model. The new reimbursement strategy was part of Geisinger's ProvenCare program, which focused on services related to elective coronary artery bypass graft (CABG) surgery. Through ProvenCare, the Geisinger team set a single price for all care associated with CABG surgery, including complications up to 90 days post surgery. This "warranty"[2] offered payers protection against costs associated with complications following heart surgery, and gave providers strong incentive to avoid complications.

Realigning payment incentives led to reengineering of this elective bypass surgery. To achieve this, Geisinger standardized care processes and workflows, enhanced the functionality of their electronic medical records to support consistency (e.g., by automating reminders), and added a "patient compact" to engage patients in personal health management. The patient compact included commitments from ProvenCare patients to: (1) communicate with providers as a team; (2) involve the patient's family and loved ones; (3) complete important care steps; and (4) improve health and prevention. In addition, Geisinger embedded 40 best-practice processes into its clinical system for delivery of care to elective CABG surgery patients (see Appendix A).

In less than a year, ProvenCare raised compliance with all 40 evidence-based care protocols from 59 percent of cases to 100 percent of cases.[3] Research published by Dr. Alfred Casale, Chief of Cardiothoracic Surgery at Geisinger, found additional benefits in decreased hospital charges and length of stay.[4]

Building on its success with episode-based payment for CABG patients, Geisinger designed a payment and delivery reform model for primary care, known as the ProvenHealth Navigator (PHN). Geisinger implemented its PHN for Medicare Advantage enrollees in 11 pilot sites across the system. Their goal was straightforward: "to prevent illness and keep people out of the hospital."[5] (The reader will readily see how difficult this strategy would be financially for a hospital, in the absence of payment reform.)

The PHN model was designed with five central components: (1) patient-centered primary care team practices; (2) integrated population management; (3) high-value referral networks; (4) quality outcomes programs; and (5) value-based reimbursement.[6] In the PHN pilot, Geisinger provided two payments to the pilot practices: a monthly payment of $1,800 per physician and a monthly stipend of $5,000 per 1,000 Medicare members to the pilot physician practice to cover additional costs of care and resources. Monthly payments to the pilot sites are paid in addition to ongoing fee-for-service reimbursement for billable services. Practice stipends are used to fund activities that are not traditionally billable, such as care coordination.

In addition, Geisinger rewarded the pilot practices using a shared-savings approach (akin to the new Medicare Accountable Care Organization program), allocating the difference between actual and expected costs among physicians and their support teams. To assure that providers lower the cost of care through improving care coordination and eliminating duplicative or unnecessary services, and not by reducing access or quality, Geisinger conditions the shared savings payments for providers on ten measures of high-quality care.

Medical claims data under the PHN model show a total cumulative reduction by 18 percent of inpatient admissions, or 56 fewer admissions per 1,000 members per year. This was accompanied by a reduction in readmission rates. **The difference attributable to PHN was 21 fewer readmissions per 1,000 members per year, or approximately a 36 percent reduction.**[7] In a survey for patients and providers regarding their experience in PHN, Geisinger found that 72 percent of patient respondents answered yes when asked if the quality of care is different and better than the past, while 86 percent of provider respondents agreed that PHN has allowed them to provide more comprehensive care than the previous system.[8]

Through its ProvenCare initiatives, Geisinger has demonstrated how payment reform mechanisms can drive quality and efficiency and improve provider and patient experiences within our health care system.

Priority Area II: Primary and Preventive Care

The primary and preventative care provisions in the Affordable Care Act (ACA) seek to shift away from a "sick care" system toward one that prevents sickness from happening in the first place.[i] Beyond the ACA, numerous public and private efforts seek to improve outcomes and curb spending by prioritizing preventative and community-based care. One of the leading efforts, the Vermont Blueprint for Health, demonstrates the potential of prevention-based primary care delivery.

Vermont Blueprint for Health

In 2006, the Vermont legislature passed Act 191, which created the Vermont Blueprint for Health. As the program has expanded, its "Triple Aim" has remained to improve health care and health services for individuals, improve population health, and improve control over rising health care costs. The Blueprint calls for the formation of Advanced Primary Care Practices (APCP) to serve as patient-centered medical homes[ii] alongside locally-based Community Health Teams (CHTs), which support and coordinate care for patients in APCPs. Pilot programs are centered around CHTs and are supported by a statewide information technology (IT) infrastructure to retain data on health information and quality improvement.

Community Health Teams

Currently, three Vermont CHTs serve approximately 49,000 residents in the St. Johnsbury, Burlington, and Barre areas. Each team is comprised of approximately five full-time-equivalent employees, which typically include nurse coordinators, behavioral health counselors, and social workers. The needs of the local patient population determine the team's composition. In St. Johnsbury, for example, the CHT includes a care integration manager, a registered nurse, several part-time behavioral health specialists, and a community health worker. Other types of practitioners are employed by the CHTs in Burlington and Barre, including social workers, dieticians, discharge coordinators, and counselors. Private insurers and the State's Medicaid program fund the CHTs with annual payments so that patients who are enrolled in an APCP receive CHT services free of charge.

---

[i] See Patient Protection and Affordable Care Act (Pub. L. 111-148) §§ 2602, 2703, 3024, 3026, 3146, 3502, 3503, 4001, 4108, 4201, 4202, 5604, and 10333. (2010).

[ii] In 2003, the Rhode Island Department of Health, in partnership with the American Academy of Pediatrics of Rhode Island, the Rhode Island Parent Information Network/Family Voices, and Neighborhood Health Plan of Rhode Island, established a medical home initiative for children with special health care needs (CSHCN) and their families, called the Pediatric Practice Enhancement Project (PPEP). PPEP places specially-trained parents of CSHCN in pediatric primary and specialty care sites across the state to serve as Family Resource Specialists and promote a medical home among families, pediatric practices, and community resources. A 2009 evaluation by the Rhode Island Department of Health found that PPEP has significantly improved care for CSHCN, including lowering PPEP participants' inpatient utilization by 24 percent compared to pre-PPEP and 34 percent compared to CSHCN in standard care. The program also lowered annual health care costs for PPEP participants by 39 percent compared to pre-PPEP and 27 percent compared to CSHCN in standard care. For more information see: Silow-Carroll, S. (2010). *Rhode Island's pediatric practice enhancement project: parents helping parents and practitioners*. Retrieved March 2012, from The Commonwealth Fund: http://www.commonwealthfund.org/~/media/Files/Publications/Case%20Study/2010/Jan/1361_SilowCarroll_Rhode_Island_PPEP_case_study.pdf.

CHTs provide care coordination, preventive health services, and improve personal health management. The teams also help patients overcome social, economic, or behavioral barriers to improving health. Addressing these non-medical barriers is particularly important to patients with chronic diseases and mental health conditions, who are often among the 5 percent utilizing 50 percent of the costs.[9]

Identifying and assessing at-risk patients is also an important task of CHTs. Vermont's IT infrastructure allows team leaders to review patient medical records and assess gaps in recommended care. These predictive analytic tools help team leaders identify and engage patients before their conditions deteriorate. CHTs are intended to interact with patients in the community at large, rather than solely at the point of care.

Early Program Effects

In the Blueprint model, collection and evaluation of clinical and administrative data is a top priority. Researchers have conducted data evaluation, focus groups, and interviews to understand the effects CHTs are having on service areas. **A four-year review of hospital data showed substantial drops in the rate of inpatient admissions (25.1 percent) and emergency department visits (22.1 percent) among patients served by CHTs.** In addition, data from a statewide all-payer claims database (the Vermont Healthcare Claims Uniform Reporting and Evaluation System) showed that overall utilization for CHT patients declined by approximately 8.9 percent, and per member per month costs dropped by approximately 11.6 percent.[10]

Early evidence shows that community health teams' emphasis on primary care and prevention has helped improve patient outcomes and overall access to care, including access to mental health services, all while reducing the cost of providing care.

Priority Area III: Measuring and Reporting Quality

Founded in 1975, Intermountain Healthcare (Intermountain) is a not-for-profit, integrated-delivery health care system that provides care to residents of Utah and southeastern Idaho. The Intermountain system is made up of 23 hospitals, approximately 160 clinics, and more than 30,000 employees. In addition, Intermountain operates a health insurance plan, SelectHealth, and a physician practice group.

Measuring and Reporting Quality

Intermountain began systematically measuring and reporting quality in 1986.[iii] Initial results led to a critical insight: treatment variation within Intermountain – even after accounting for differences in patient diagnoses and complexity – was enormous.

In 1990, Intermountain launched the Institute for Health Care Delivery Research to further analyze practice variation and develop best practices. The Institute's data on patient satisfaction, outcomes, cost, and processes of care enabled researchers to develop evidenced-based care process models (EB-CPM).

In 1991, Alan Morris, a pulmonologist at Intermountain, introduced a care protocol at Intermountain for the treatment of acute respiratory distress syndrome. Morris's care protocol proved effective; practice variation reduced from 59 to 6 percent while survival rates rose for the sickest patients from 9.5 to 44 percent. These results occurred just four months after the protocol was introduced to the pilot hospital.

Intermountain researchers found that 104 processes accounted for almost 95 percent of the clinical care provided to patients. The success of Morris' care protocol led Intermountain to begin a system-wide expansion of these methods to all 104 care processes identified by the researchers.

Intermountain now tracks hospitals and physicians to measure and report on quality. Each month, hospitals receive summary reports that track performance against uniform benchmarks and goals. Physicians are also tracked at random each quarter and sent report cards that summarize individual performance in a particular clinical area. The goal of internal data review is to help physicians, hospitals, and other providers in Intermountain's system meet the internally-set performance benchmarks; the transparency and accountability encourages innovation and improvement.

Costs Savings and Positive Results

Intermountain has demonstrated cost savings resulting from its efforts on quality measurement and improvement. For example, Intermountain's EB-CPM for hip replacement reduced cost more than $4,000 per case in just two years. The providers within Intermountain piloting the first 65 care process models realized savings of approximately $30

---

iii In 2005, the Rhode Island Quality Institute, Quality Partners of Rhode Island (now Healthcentric Advisors), the Hospital Association of Rhode Island, the State's 11 acute care hospitals, Blue Cross & Blue Shield of Rhode Island, and United Healthcare of New England launched a statewide quality improvement initiative called the Rhode Island Intensive Care Unit (ICU) Collaborative. The goals of the ICU Collaborative are to improve the culture of safety and clinical outcomes for central line-associated blood stream infections (CLABSI), ventilator-associated pneumonia (VAP), sepsis, and palliative care in Rhode Island's adult ICUs. As part of the Collaborative, a web-based data collection tool was created to enable hospitals to report collected data on ICU infections in "real time," and a program to educate health care workers on best practice strategies for reducing complications from the conditions listed above was implemented. Rhode Island is the only state in the nation to achieve 100 percent hospital participation in such a program. The most recent data show that Rhode Island's ICU Collaborative reduced CLABSI and VAP rates by 61 percent and 7.8 percent respectively, resulting in an estimated 97 lives, 4,415 hospital days and nearly $13 million saved. Sepsis mortality has also declined by approximately 16 percent, resulting in an additional estimate of 43 lives saved. For more information, see: McNicoll, L., DePalo, V., Cornell, M., Rocha, J., & Adams, L. (2009). *The Rhode Island ICU Collaborative: The first statewide collaborative four years later. Medicine & Health/Rhode Island*, 92(8). Retrieved from http://www.rimed.org/medhealthri/2009-08/2009-08-273.pdf.

million in less than ten years. Had the process models been applied system-wide, savings could have reached $100 million, or approximately six percent of clinical costs. **In 2008, researchers from the Dartmouth Atlas Project estimated that the United States could reduce health care spending by more than 40 percent if all providers adopted the practices of Intermountain Healthcare.**[11]

Intermountain provided testimony to the HELP Committee last year demonstrating its continuing commitment to reducing costs by improving the quality of care for its patients, and its confidence that its experience can be replicated system-wide.

Priority Area IV: Administrative Simplification

Effective administrative simplification demands multi-stakeholder buy-in, as well as public-private effort, since standardized administrative process reforms cross the health care spectrum. This section examines administrative reforms enacted across the public and private sector in four broad areas: (1) simplification of provider credentialing; (2) improvements in health care insurance eligibility processes; (3) standardization of health insurance identification cards; and (4) standardization of prior authorization (PA) processes.[12] The Healthcare Administrative Simplification Coalition (HASC) highlights these priority areas and further identifies potential savings in the order of billions of dollars each year.[13]

Provider Credentialing

Provider credentialing is an administrative process ideally suited for reducing costs and wasteful duplication of effort. Health plans and provider organizations, including hospitals, are required by law to verify physician credentials to ensure that physicians meet minimum standards for licensure and competency before they are given hospital privileges or included in networks. Streamlining this process presents an opportunity to reduce the time and resources providers and other entities devote to credentialing.

An online data model to simplify the credentialing process already exists: the Universal Provider Datasource (UPD). Since its 2002 launch, UPD provides more than 960,000 physician credentials to more than 600 health plans and providers.[14] The benefits of this system include uniform collection of credentialing requirements, reduction in process repetition and errors, and decreased operating costs.

In 2004, the Medical Group Management Association (MGMA) analyzed the effects of a streamlined credentialing process. MGMA found that early cost savings across health entities reached $92 million per year or, equivalently, 1,500 full-time employees each year.[15] The Council for Affordable Quality Healthcare (CAQH) estimates system-wide savings between $150 million and $200 million if UPD were deployed across the health care system. A similar estimate

developed by the UnitedHealth Group (UHG) forecast national savings from unified provider credentialing of about $18 billion — $10 billion of which would accrue to providers — over the next decade.[16]

Eligibility Verification and Claims Processing

Claims processing and patient eligibility verification generate waste due to variation in payment processes across payers. Despite mandated electronic data interchange (EDI) standards, there is limited adoption of automated processes that could yield substantial efficiencies in provider billing and payment. As a result, the CAQH Committee on Operating Rules for Information Exchange (CORE) developed a set of operating rules to enhance interoperability; streamline eligibility, benefits, and claims transactions; and reduce the amount of time and resources spent on administrative functions.[17]

A recent study conducted by IBM Global Business Services studied the effects of the CORE operating rules across 6 health plans, 33 million Americans, 5 clearinghouses/vendors, and 6 providers. Overall, the CORE operating rules reduced administrative costs and increased utilization of health information technology. Health plans, on average, saved $2.6 million each year after implementation. Providers experienced a 10-12 percent decrease in claims denials as well as a reduction in accounts receivable.[18] Providers verified 24 percent more patients and saved $2.60 per electronic verification.[19] IBM projects that standardized operating rules will save $4.60 per transaction. With an estimated 1.3 billion eligibility verifications each year, the transaction savings resulting from standardized operating rules could be considerable.[20]

Health Insurance Identification Cards

Inconsistency among health insurance identification cards presents another opportunity for reform. Uniform health identification cards, with magnetic stripes that store this information electronically, convey accurate patient and plan information to providers at the point of service and reduce claim denials, administrative errors, and processing time.

UnitedHealth Group (UHG) has introduced 30 million cards to plan members, and early benefits include ease of use for the consumer, support of electronic eligibility verification, and identification of accurate copayment at the time care is delivered. Despite challenges and barriers to adoption, UHG estimates savings of $18 million over the next ten years.

Prior Authorization

The prior authorization (PA) process is highly complex, and the requirements vary from one entity to the next. Providers and plans would benefit from a process that is more transparent and automated; clinicians could reduce the amount of time they spend on preauthorization and increase time spent on care. In one survey of physician practices, prior authorization was reported to be the second most time-consuming activity associated with managing insurance company-related tasks (compliance with formularies was the first).[21] Recognizing the opportunity to streamline prior authorization, in 2009 the Minnesota legislature required the Department of Health produce guidelines to standardize prior authorization requests by providers for prescription drugs. Accordingly, the Department of Health produced a uniform form intended for electronic submission. The law also requires that all prior authorization requests be "accessible and submitted by health care providers, and accepted by group purchasers, electronically through secure electronic transmissions" by January 1, 2015.[22]

System efficiency can be enhanced by administrative simplification, and the four key focus areas cited above identify opportunity for substantial improvements. Across the continuum of care, organizations would benefit from innovative solutions that consistently standardize, simplify, and automate system transactions so that benefits exceed costs.

Priority Area V: Health Information Technology

Founded in 1916, the Marshfield Clinic is a multi-specialty group practice that provides care to residents of Wisconsin. The clinic is a not-for-profit organization that employs over 775 physicians and 6,600 support staff across 54 locations. Each practice site is "fully electronic, paperless, and linked by common information systems."[23] Every year, the system encounters more than 3.8 million visits and treats over 375,000 patients from predominantly rural communities, often through a regional ambulatory care system made of 41 care sites. The Marshfield Clinic also owns and operates Security Health Plan of Wisconsin (SHP), a physician-sponsored health maintenance organization covering over 175,000 members.

Marshfield Clinic's Excellence with Information Technology

To achieve its mission and practice goals, the Clinic has made continued investments in information technology (IT) systems.[iv] In 1985, the Clinic developed an extensive electronic medical record (EMR), commonly referred to as CattailsMD, to document patient information. Rather than including medical information strictly from new patient encounters, the Clinic decided to input data for all patients dating as far back as 1960.

Marshfield physicians and support staff use the EMR to access patient information on diagnoses, treatment plans, procedures, medication lists, laboratory and imaging results, and clinical notes, among other items. CattailsMD also supports additional analytic and reporting functionalities, such as built-in decision support. [24] Decision support facilitates safe and appropriate care with patient-specific prompts and checkpoints to reduce harmful drug interactions and prescribing errors (e.g. allergies). The EMR also improves the efficiency of clinical operations by giving physicians real-time access to test, laboratory, or imaging results. Moreover, CattailsMD strengthens primary care services through chronic disease and preventive care registries.

The Clinic also uses its IT systems to support telemedicine services (particularly critical for its rural population).[25, 26] Marshfield Clinic TeleHealth improves patient care with a three-pronged approach that: (1) links clinicians to each other; (2) links patients to clinicians; and (3) transfers medical information. Doctors and patients can connect via phone lines or through conferencing services that enable face-to-face interactions for clinical or educational purposes. The Clinic's most notable telemedicine program is for anticoagulation services to telephonically monitor patients who take the drug Coumadin.

Proven Success of Information Technology at the Marshfield Clinic

Costs savings associated with the IT-supported delivery model at the Marshfield Clinic have been captured in several ways. First, results from the Physician Group Practice (PGP) Demonstration indicate that Marshfield experienced improvements in clinical performance. In a prior study conducted by the Agency for Healthcare Research and Quality, patients in Marshfield Clinic's anticoagulation program had lower hospitalization rates and adverse events when compared to patients receiving routine care. Internal researchers from the Clinic found that Medicare beneficiaries who participated in the anticoagulant pilot program had nearly 29 fewer hospitalizations per 100 persons per year. **The reduction in the hospitalization rate amounted to savings of approximately $271,014 per 100 persons per year.**[27]

Marshfield also realized savings as a result of its paperless culture. PGP demonstration researchers found that physicians saved considerable time by using the EMR. On average, physicians saved between three to seven minutes per

---

iv In 2005, Blue Cross & Blue Shield of Rhode Island launched its "Quality Counts" program: a five-year pilot program designed to increase the use of electronic health records, transform the way care is delivered, and improve quality of care. Through the pilot, 79 primary care physicians received partial funding for the purchase of an electronic health record system and monthly stipends in the first and second year of the program to compensate for time spent on electronic health record implementation and workflow redesign activities. Participating physicians also had the opportunity to receive performance bonus dollars based on improved preventive care and outcomes for 10 quality measures established by BCBSRI in conjunction with participating primary care physicians. At the end of the program, BCBSRI reported improved health quality measures, with median improvement rates of 44 percent in family and children's health metrics, 35 percent in women's care metrics, and 24 percent in internal medicine metrics. All 79 of the participating physicians successfully implemented electronic health records. The "Quality Counts" program has served as the foundation for BCBSRI's Patient-Centered Medical Home program, which currently includes more than 25 percent of Rhode Island's primary care physicians. For more information see http://www.bcbs.com/why-bcbs/health-reform/pathway.pdf.

visit. In aggregate, this amounts to approximately 200 to 466 additional hours per physician per year.[28]

Since going paperless in 2007, the Marshfield Clinic has achieved annual savings of about $7 million as a result of consolidating space and job functionality.[29] Moreover, improved clinical processes generate cost savings. For example, the electronic prescribing function discussed above encourages "preferred alternatives" for drug choice, saving more than $2.5 million in one year through the substitution of higher-cost with lower-cost drugs.[30] The EMR at Marshfield also generates administrative cost savings by streamlining transactions between the Clinic and payers, which decreases claim denials. At Marshfield, claims are denied less than two percent of the time.[31]

Conclusion

Despite ongoing challenges posed by misaligned payment incentives and infrastructure gaps (e.g., the lack of health information exchange capabilities), these examples represent a growing number of successful delivery system reform models. The strategies within the ACA to encourage broader efforts at system transformation show real promise. Numerous other projects demonstrate similar success, and reinforce the promise of delivery system innovation: to save patients lives and families worry, while saving taxpayer, business, and individual pocketbook dollars. It is in this context that we proceed to evaluate the implementation by the Obama Administration of the ACA delivery system reform sections, and whether the diligence and focus of that effort is commensurate with the promise of the reform path.

ENDNOTES

1   Paulus, R., Davis, K., & Steele, G. (2008). Continuous innovation in health care: Implications of the Geisinger experience. *Health Affairs, 27*(5), 1235-1245.

2   Abelson, R. (2007, May 17). In bid for better hospital care, heart surgery with a warranty. *New York Times*. Retrieved from http://www.nytimes.com/2007/05/17/business/17quality.html

3   Casale, A., Paulus, R., Selna, M., Doll, M., Bothe, A., McKinley, K., . . . Steele, G. (2007). "ProvenCareSM": A provider-driven pay-for-performance program for acute episodic cardiac surgical care. *Annals of Surgery, 246*(4), 613-623.

4   Ibid.

5   Geisinger - Innovations Loader. Retrieved February 15, 2012 from http://www.geisinger.org/innovations/index.html

6   Gilfillan, R., Tomcavage, J., Rosenthal, M., Davis, D., Graham, J., Roy, J., Pierdon, S., . . . Steele, G. (2010). Value and the medical home: Effects of transformed primary care. *American Journal of Managed Care, 16*(8), 607-614.

7   Ibid.

8   Geisinger Health System. (2011).

9   Cohen, S. & Yu, W. (2012). *The concentration and persistence in the level of health expenditures over time: Estimates for the U.S. population, 2007-2008*. Agency for Healthcare Research and Quality, Statistical Brief No. 354. Retrieved from http://meps.ahrq.gov/mepsweb/data_files/publications/st354/stat354.pdf

10   Department of Vermont Health Access. (2011). *Vermont Blueprint for Health: 2010 Annual report*. Retrieved from http://hcr.vermont.gov/sites/hcr/files/final_annual_report_01_26_11.pdf

11   Dartmouth Institute for Health Policy & Clinical Practice. (2008) *An agenda for change: Improving quality and curbing health care spending: Opportunities for the Congress and the Obama Administration*. Retrieved from http://www.dartmouthatlas.org/downloads/reports/agenda_for_change.pdf

12   Ibid.

13   Ibid.

14   Council for Affordable Quality Healthcare. *Universal provider datasource*. Retrieved on February 15, 2012 from http://www.caqh.org/ucd.php

15   The Healthcare Administrative Simplification Coalition. (2009). *Bringing better value: Recommendations to address the costs and causes of administrative complexity in the nation's healthcare system*. Retrieved from http://www.ahima.org/downloads/pdfs/advocacy/HASCReport20090717.pdf

16   UnitedHealth Center for Health Reform & Modernization. (2009). *Health care cost containment — How technology can cut red tape and simplify health care administration*. Minneapolis: UnitedHealth Group. Retrieved on February 15, 2012 from http://www.unitedhealthgroup.com/hrm/unh_workingpaper2.pdf

17   Council for Affordable Quality Healthcare. *CORE overview: Simplifying healthcare administration*. Retrieved on February 9, 2012 from http://caqh.org/CORE_overview.php

18   Council for Affordable Quality Healthcare. (2009, May). *CAQH CORE phase I measures of success executive summary and industry-wide savings projection*. Retrieved from http://www.caqh.org/pdf/COREIBMstudy.pdf

19   Ibid.

20   Ibid.

21   Casalino, L., Nicholson, S., Gans, D., Hammons, T., Morra, D., Karrison, T., Levinson, W. (2009). What does it cost physician practices to interact with health insurance plans? *Health Affairs, 28*(4), w533-w543.

22   Minnesota Department of Health. (2010, February 15). *Electronic drug prior authorization standardization and transmission: Report to the Minnesota legislature 2010*. Retrieved from http://www.health.state.mn.us/asa/rxpa021510rpt.pdf

23   Ulrich, K. (2009, June 25). Testimony on health care reform before the Health Subcommittee of the Committee on Energy and Commerce, U.S. House of Representatives, Washington, DC. Retrieved from http://www.marshfieldclinic.org/proxy/MC-Ulrich-testimony.1.pdf

24   Ibid.

25   Antoniotti, N. (2005). Telethinking with Nina M. Antoniotti. *Telemedicine Journal and E-Health, 11*(5), 517-521.

26   Antoniotti, N. (2007, May). *TeleHealth and EMRs: Talking the telehealth language*. Presented at the annual meeting of the American Telemedicine Association. Nashville, TN.

27   Hillman, M. (2002, April 16). Testimony before the Subcommittee on Health of the Committee on Ways and Means, U.S. House of Representatives, Washington, DC. Retrieved from http://www.gpo.gov/fdsys/pkg/CHRG-107hhrg82324/html/CHRG-107hhrg82324.htm

28   Microsoft Global Evidence Management System. (2004). *Healthcare clinic saves money and improves quality of care with Tablet PC solution*. (Customer Solution Case Study). Redmond, WA.

29   McCarthy, D., Mueller, K., & Klein, S. (2009). *Marshfield Clinic: Health information technology paves the way for population health management*. New York: Commonwealth Fund.

30   Ibid.

31   CattailsMD, electronic medical record (EMR) and practice management system. Marshfield, WI: Marshfield Clinic Information Systems. Retrieved on February 15, 2012 from http://www.cattailssoftware.com/?page=cattails-products-cattailsmd

CHAPTER FOUR

Status of Federal Delivery System Reform Implementation

The Affordable Care Act (ACA) supports the transformation of health care delivery in the United States through numerous, interconnected reforms. This chapter examines the scope of, and progress toward, implementation of delivery system reform pursuant to the ACA. To do so, we identify provisions of the law that influence the structure and performance of health care delivery. Our analysis targets policies that alter the incentives, information, or obligations of health care providers. This includes demonstration and pilot programs that test new delivery models, as well as policies that improve operational aspects of health care delivery, such as standardization of forms and electronic processes and coordination of federal and state policies.

Using these criteria, we identified 45 delivery system reforms that are the subject of this chapter. Appendix B lists the reform provisions, organized by the five priority areas described earlier in the report: (1) payment reform; (2) primary and preventive care; (3) measuring and reporting quality; (4) administrative simplification; and (5) health information technology. Areas of the law not included in this report are provisions that govern coverage expansion, health insurance exchanges, regulation of insurance, and benefit design. In addition, Medicare and Medicaid payment provisions not associated with changes in payment methods or tied to other delivery reforms are not reviewed in this report.

The Affordable Care Act created a wide array of new responsibilities for the Department of Health and Human Services (HHS). The law states the "Secretary shall" 1,099 times. Of those 1,099 directives, at least 290 appear in the 45 delivery system reform provisions described in Appendix B. The Secretary of HHS oversees the implementation of the delivery system reforms described in Appendix B. Often, specific tasks within a section of the law are assigned to, delegated, or worked on in conjunction with agencies or bureaus within HHS and its component agencies. For example, §3013, Quality Measure Development, requires the Secretary to consult with the Administrator of the Centers for Medicare & Medicaid Services (CMS) and the Director of the Agency for Healthcare Research and Quality (AHRQ) to identify gaps in quality measurement and develop new quality measures.

Each "Secretary Shall" defines a set of tasks that must be unpacked, delegated to offices and agencies within HHS, and coordinated and monitored by the Secretary's office. These tasks include, but are not limited to, establishing new entities and advisory groups, awarding grants and contracts, conducting evaluations, submitting reports to Congress, establishing demonstration projects and pilot programs, collecting data and information, rulemaking, soliciting provider participation and input, and establishing oversight and monitoring systems.

In this chapter, we review the Administration's progress implementing the law's delivery system reform provisions within the five priority areas. For each provision, we describe the law's intent, review the steps taken toward implementation, and note the extent to which deadlines (when applicable) have and have not been met.

The provisions below are listed in the order in which they appear in the Affordable Care Act. This format does not reflect a provision's priority level or importance, its breadth, and/or its potential affect on the health care system. However, we expect certain provisions to have a further-reaching effect on transforming the delivery of care than others. For example, under payment reform, these include the Center for Medicare and Medicaid Innovation (§3021), the Hospital Value-Based Purchasing Program (§3001(a)), the Medicare Shared Savings Program (§3022), and the Payment Adjustments for Hospital and Health Care-Acquired Conditions (§3008; §2702). In the primary and preventive care section, such provisions include the Coverage and Payment for Dual Eligibles (§2602), the Community-based Care Transitions Program (§3026), and the Community Transformation Grants (§4201). Within each priority area, there are provisions with higher degrees of significance and potential to create change in our health care system. It is important to keep this in mind when evaluating the Administration's implementation effort.

Priority Area 1: Payment Reform

In this section, we highlight 15 ACA provisions that primarily concern payment reform. These include:

1. Medicaid Payment Adjustment for Health Care-Acquired Conditions (§2702);
2. Medicaid Bundled Payment Demonstration (§2704);
3. Medicaid Global Payment System Demonstration Project (§2705);
4. Medicaid Pediatric Accountable Care Organization Demonstration Program (§2706);
5. Medicaid Emergency Psychiatric Demonstration Project (§2707);
6. Hospital Value-Based Purchasing Program (§3001(a));
7. Value-Based Purchasing Demonstration Programs (§3001(b));
8. Value-Based Purchasing Programs for Skilled Nursing Facilities, Home Health Agencies, and Ambulatory Surgical Centers (§3006; §10301);
9. Physician Value-Based Payment Modifier (§3007);
10. Hospital-Acquired Condition Payment Adjustment (§3008);

11. Center for Medicare and Medicaid Innovation (§3021);
12. Medicare Shared Savings Program (§3022);
13. National Medicare Payment Bundling Pilot Program (§3023);
14. Hospital Readmission Reduction Program (§3025); and
15. The Independent Payment Advisory Board (§3403).

Overall, seven of the 15 provisions have been implemented; one provision is partially complete (see the note below); three policies have not been implemented, but are not yet overdue; three demonstration projects for which funds have not been appropriated have not been launched by the timelines detailed in the law; and two reports to Congress – the value-based purchasing implementation plan for skilled nursing facilities (due October 1, 2011) and the report on expanding hospital-acquired conditions penalties (due January 1, 2012) – are delayed. Both of these reports are in the final review process within the Administration.

§2702 (Medicaid Payment Adjustment for Health-Care-Acquired Conditions) requires the Secretary to identify state policies that prohibit payment for health-care-acquired conditions and issue regulations prohibiting federal Medicaid payment to states for certain health-care-acquired conditions. The law requires the regulations be effective as of July 1, 2011. On June 6, 2011, CMS published a final rule prohibiting Medicaid payment for a set of health care-acquired conditions. The final rule was effective July 1, 2011. CMS is allowing states until July 1, 2012 to comply with the final regulation.

§2704 (Medicaid Bundled Payment Demonstration Project) establishes a five-year demonstration project in up to eight states to study the use of bundled payments for hospital and physician services in Medicaid. The demonstration project was required to begin on January 1, 2012. The law also requires a report to Congress one year after the conclusion of the demonstration project. The demonstration project does not include appropriation of implementation funding specific to it and no funds for implementation have been identified. Due to these factors, work on §2704 has not been initiated. At a minimum, funding for staffing and evaluation of the project is necessary to begin plans for implementation.

§2705 (Medicaid Global Payment System Demonstration Project) establishes a demonstration project for FY2010 through FY2012 under which up to five states would adjust their Medicaid payment model for eligible safety-net hospital systems or networks. Instead of fee-for-service payment, states would switch to a global, capitated-payment model for safety-net hospitals. The CMS Innovation Center is required to test and evaluate this demonstration project to examine any changes in health care quality outcomes and spending by the eligible safety-net hospital systems or networks. One year after the completion of the demonstra-

tion project, the Secretary is required to submit a report to Congress that includes the results to the Innovation Center's evaluation and recommendations for legislation and administrative action. The law does not have an appropriation of funding specific to §2705, and no funds for implementation have been identified. Due to these factors, work on §2705 has not been initiated. At a minimum, funding for staffing and evaluation of the project is necessary to begin plans for implementation.

§2706 (Medicaid Pediatric Accountable Care Organization Demonstration Project) establishes a five-year demonstration project through which participating states may recognize pediatric providers as accountable care organizations (ACOs) for the purpose of receiving incentive payments associated with cost control and quality improvement. The statutory deadline for the launch of this demonstration program was January 1, 2012. The demonstration project does not include appropriation of implementation funding specific to it and no funds for implementation have been identified. Due to these factors, work on §2706 has not been initiated. At a minimum, funding for staffing and evaluation of the project is necessary to begin plans for implementation.

§2707 (Medicaid Emergency Psychiatric Demonstration Project) requires the Secretary to establish a competitive, three-year demonstration project under which eligible states will provide payment under its State Medicaid plan to an "institution for mental diseases" for providing medical assistance to individuals who are between the ages 21 and 65, are eligible for Medicaid, and require medical attention for an emergency medical condition. The Secretary is required to evaluate the demonstration project's effect on access to inpatient mental health services and cost, and provide a recommendation on whether the project should be continued after 2013 and expanded nationally. The Secretary must also submit a report to Congress, not later than December 31, 2013, on the findings of the evaluation previously described. On March 13, 2012, CMS announced that 11 States and the District of Columbia will participate in the Medicaid Emergency Psychiatric Demonstration, including Alabama, California, Connecticut, Illinois, Maine, Maryland, Missouri, North Carolina, Rhode Island, Washington, and West Virginia.

§3001(a) (Hospital Value-Based Purchasing Program) establishes a Medicare value-based purchasing (VBP) program under Medicare for hospitals starting in FY2013. The value-based incentive payments will be based on hospital performance on quality measures related to high-cost conditions and measures of patients' care experience. By law, the Secretary is required to take several actions to establish the VBP program including, among other actions, developing methodologies for evaluating hospital performance, establishing performance standards, and submitting a report to Congress by January 1, 2016. The Secretary is also required to promulgate regulations to carry out the program. On May 6, 2011, CMS published a final rule to implement the hospital VBP program. Other hospital VBP measures were published in the Federal Register on August 18, 2011.

§3001(b) (Value-Based Purchasing Demonstration Programs) establishes two, three-year value-based purchasing demonstration programs under Medicare. The demonstration programs are intended to: (1) test innovative methods of measuring and rewarding efficient health care services at inpatient, critical access hospitals; and (2) test VBP for hospitals excluded from the VBP program established under §3001(a) due to insufficient number of measures and cases. For both demonstration programs, the Secretary is required to submit a report (18 months after the completion of the demonstration programs) to Congress with recommendations to permanently establish VBP programs for these types of hospitals. The demonstration programs were to be established not later than March 23, 2012. To date, no funds for implementation have been identified and work on the demonstrations has not been initiated.

§3006 as amended by §10301(a) (Value-Based Purchasing Program for Skilled Nursing Facilities, Home Health Agencies, and Ambulatory Surgical Centers) requires the Secretary to develop a plan to implement a Medicare VBP program for skilled nursing facilities, home health agencies, and ambulatory surgical centers. The Secretary must submit a report to Congress about the plan for implementing a VBP program for skilled nursing facilities and home health agencies (by Oct. 1, 2011) and ambulatory surgical centers (by January 1, 2011). This provision is partially complete. CMS released reports to Congress on the VBP implementation plan for ambulatory surgical centers and home health agencies, but the report for skilled nursing facilities has not been released. It is in the process of final review within the Administration.

§3007 (Physician Value-based Payment Modifier) requires the Secretary to develop and implement a budget-neutral, pay-for-performance program for physicians based on the quality and cost of care they deliver. The law requires the quality and cost measures to be risk-adjusted and standardized within geographic regions. There are several deadlines associated with this provision. The Secretary was required to publish quality measures and costs, dates for implementation of the payment modifier, and the performance period by January 1, 2012. HHS must begin implementing the payment modifier through a rulemaking process in 2013. Beginning January 1, 2015, the Secretary must apply the payment modifier to select physicians and physician groups. Finally, not later than January 1, 2017, the Secretary must apply the modifier to all physicians and groups of physicians. On November 28, 2011, HHS published the measures for quality of care and cost for the physician value-based payment

modifier in the Federal Register. In the rule, CMS identified CY2013 as the performance year for purposes of adjusting physician payments in CY2015.

§3008 (Hospital-Acquired Condition Payment Adjustment) establishes penalties for hospitals with rates for certain hospital-acquired conditions (HACs) in the top quartile. Penalties are scheduled to begin in FY2015. The law requires the Secretary to determine if penalties should be extended to other providers including nursing homes, inpatient rehabilitations facilities, long-term care hospitals, outpatient hospital departments, ambulatory surgical centers, and health clinics. A report to Congress on expanding HAC penalties to non-hospital providers was due on January 1, 2012. HHS is in the process of finalizing the report.

§3021 (Center for Medicare and Medicaid Innovation) was established by the ACA to identify, develop, support and evaluate payment and service delivery models for Medicare and Medicaid. The law provides the Innovation Center authority to implement new models of care delivery quickly, and encourage the widespread adoption of practices that prove to deliver better health at lower cost. The Innovation Center was established in 2011, and has implemented 13 initiatives to test and disseminate new payment models and other delivery system reforms. These initiatives include:

- the Federally-Qualified Health Center Advanced Primary Care Practice Demonstration;
- the Pioneer ACO Model;
- the Advanced Payment ACO Model;
- Bundled Payments for Care Improvement;
- the Comprehensive Primary Care Initiative;
- State Demonstrations to Integrate Care for Dual Eligible Individuals;
- Financial Models to Support State Efforts to Integrate Care for Medicare and Medicaid Beneficiaries;
- Initiative to Reduce Avoidable Hospitalizations among Nursing Facility Residents;
- Partnership for Patients;
- the Health Care Innovation Challenge;
- the Innovation Advisors Program;
- Million Hearts; and
- Strong Start for Mothers and Newborns.

The ACA gives the Secretary of HHS the authority to expand successful pilots supported and evaluated by the Innovation Center through the rulemaking process (rather than requiring new legislation) if doing so is expected to reduce spending or improve the quality of care and the Chief Actuary of CMS certifies that such expansion would reduce program spending. While the Secretary has yet to use the rulemaking authority, we expect this mechanism should speed the adoption of evidence-based policy reforms in Medicare and Medicaid.

§3022 (Medicare Shared Savings Program) establishes a shared savings program, not later than January 1, 2012, in which providers can opt to work as accountable care organizations (ACOs) to manage and coordinate care for Medicare beneficiaries. In the ACO arrangement, providers accept accountability for both the quality of care and total spending for a population of Medicare beneficiaries. Providers are eligible to receive shared savings payments if the average per capita Medicare expenditure under the ACO is less than the benchmark established by the Secretary. On November 2, 2011, the Secretary published final regulations outlining the Medicare Shared Savings program for ACOs. The regulation established criteria for participation, including primary care capacity, quality measurement obligations, and governance requirements.

§3023 (National Medicare Payment Bundling Pilot Program) establishes a five-year, voluntary pilot program encouraging hospitals, doctors, and post-acute care providers to improve patient care and achieve savings for Medicare through bundled payments. The pilot is expected to begin January 1, 2013. Not later than January 1, 2016, the Secretary is required to submit an implementation plan to Congress about expanding the pilot program. To date, no funds for implementation have been identified and work on the pilot program has not been initiated.

§3025 (Hospital Readmission Reduction Program) introduces a downward payment adjustment for inpatient stays that reflects the hospital's percentage readmission rate for heart attack, heart failure, and pneumonia admissions. The payment adjustment takes effect in FY2013 for hospital discharges on or after October 1, 2012. The law also authorizes the Secretary to expand the readmission adjustment to other conditions beginning in FY2015, and make hospital readmission rates public. On August 18, 2011, CMS issued a final rule on the measures and methodology to calculate excess readmission rates (the rule was part of the Medicare inpatient hospital payment policies and rates for FY2012).

§3403 (Independent Payment Advisory Board (IPAB)) establishes the Independent Medicare Advisory Board, an independent, 15-member commission tasked with developing proposals to address excess cost growth in any year that Medicare spending growth exceeds a target rate. Beginning January 15, 2014, the IPAB's proposals must be adopted by the Secretary unless Congress passes an alternative measure that achieves the same level of savings. The Consolidated Appropriations Act, 2012 (H.R. 2055), which was signed into law on December 23, 2011, rescinded $10 million of the $15 million appropriated by the ACA for the IPAB in FY2012. The members of the IPAB have not yet been selected, although no specific reporting deadlines have been missed.

In summary, the Administration has made significant prog-

ress implementing the payment reform provisions of the ACA, with seven of 15 provisions implemented according to legislative deadlines; one provision partially compete; three provisions not yet due to be executed; two reports to Congress overdue; and three demonstration projects that have not received funding are behind schedule. The three demonstration projects that are behind schedule involve both working in concert with State Medicaid agencies and adapting demonstration design to the widely varying financing and delivery system contexts across the country.

Priority Area 2: Primary and Preventive Care

ACA provisions that target improvements in primary and preventive care include screening and primary prevention (e.g. immunization) as well as secondary prevention and chronic disease management. From a cost control perspective, policies that target high-risk patients and prevent acute exacerbations of chronic disease are critically important.[i] We identified 14 ACA provisions that focus on primary and preventive care:

1. Coverage and Payment Coordination for Dual Eligibles (§2602);
2. Medicaid Health Home Option (§2703);
3. Medicare Independence at Home Demonstration Program (§3024);
4. Community-based Care Transitions Program (§3026);
5. Hospice Concurrent Care Demonstration Program (§3140);
6. Community Health Team Grants to Support Medical Homes (§3502);
7. Medication Therapy Management Grants (§3503);
8. National Prevention, Health Promotion, and Public Health Council (§4001);
9. Medicaid Prevention and Wellness Incentives (§4108);
10. Community Transformation Grants (§4201);
11. Community Wellness Pilot Program (§4202(a));
12. Medicare Prevention and Wellness Evaluation (§4202(b));
13. Co-Locating Primary and Specialty Care in Community-Based Mental Health Settings (§5604); and
14. Community-Based Collaborative Care Network Program (§10333).

Overall, seven of the 14 provisions have been implemented; one policy has not been implemented, but is not yet overdue; one provision for which funds have not been appropriated is overdue; and five policies have not been implemented but do not have statutory deadlines.

§2602 (Coverage and Payment Coordination for Dual Eligibles) establishes the Federal Coordinated Health Care Office not later than March 1, 2010 to improve the quality and cost-efficiency of care provided to individuals dually eligible for Medicare and Medicaid ("dual eligibles"). HHS estab-

---

i   See Patient Protection and Affordable Care Act (Pub. L. 111-148) §§ 2703, 3024, and 3026. (2010).

lished the Office and, on December 30, 2010, published a statement of the Office's organization, functions, and authority. Among other activities, the Federal Coordinated Health Care Office issued guidance to states on financing models to integrate care for dual eligibles. On April 1, 2011, the Office awarded contracts to 15 states to support innovative efforts to provide seamless Medicare and Medicaid benefits to dual eligibles, focusing on integrating acute and long-term care.

§2703 (Medicaid Health Home Option) provides states the option of enrolling Medicaid beneficiaries with chronic conditions in a "health home" (a primary care arrangement that emphasizes continuous, comprehensive, and coordinated care). The law required the Secretary to establish standards for qualification as a designated provider of health home services. On November 16, 2010, CMS issued preliminary guidance on health homes in a State Medicaid Director letter. States have had the option of electing the health home option since January 1, 2011. As of December 2011, Rhode Island and Missouri had approved State Plan Amendments with health home provisions.

§3024 (Medicare Independence at Home Demonstration Program) establishes a three-year demonstration program to test the use of primary care teams to provide services to high-need Medicare beneficiaries. Participating primary care teams will be accountable for providing comprehensive care to high-need populations at home and coordinating care across treatment settings. Like ACOs, primary care teams will be eligible to share in any savings under the demonstration program if specified quality targets are achieved. The demonstration program was due to begin by January 1, 2012. In December 2011, CMS released a solicitation inviting providers to apply for the Independence at Home Demonstration. Applications and letters of intent were due on February 6, 2012.

§3026 (Community-based Care Transitions Program) requires the Secretary to establish a five-year program to fund eligible hospitals and community-based organizations that provide evidence-based transition services to Medicare beneficiaries with multiple chronic conditions at risk for hospital readmission. The program was required to begin by January 1, 2011. On November 18, 2011, CMS announced the first seven sites to be selected for the Community-based Care Transition Program. On March 14, 2012, CMS announced 23 additional participants in the program, and will continue to accept applications for the program on a rolling basis until its dedicated funding is obligated.

§3140 (Hospice Concurrent Care Demonstration Program) directs the Secretary to establish a three-year demonstration program to examine new models for hospice care provided concurrently with other medical care. This effort is intended to address the barrier to hospice care that current Medicare policy imposes by requiring that patients choose to forgo curative (active) treatment in order to receive hospice care. The demonstration will test whether allowing patients to receive curative care alongside hospice increases use of hospice, improves patient and family outcomes, and saves Medicare resources. The demonstration program does not have an establishment date set by law. To date, no funds for implementation have been identified and work on the demonstration has not been initiated.

§3502 (Community Health Team Grants to Support Medical Homes) requires the Secretary to award grants or enter into contracts to support community-based, interdisciplinary, inter-professional health teams to support primary care medical homes. Funding is intended to support the development of health teams and to pay capitated payments to primary care providers. No deadlines are specified in the law. To date, no funds for implementation have been identified, and work on the demonstrations has not been initiated.

§3503 (Medication Therapy Management Grants) requires the Secretary to provide grants to support medication therapy management services provided by licensed pharmacists for high-risk patients. These services are intended for patients who take four or more prescribed medications, take high-risk medications, have two or more chronic diseases, or have undergone a transition of care. The grant program was expected to begin by May 1, 2010, but has not been implemented. Funding to implement these grants was authorized to come from §3501, the Patient Safety Research Center. While funding for §3501 was authorized, it has not yet been appropriated. At a minimum, funding for staffing and evaluation of the grant program is necessary to begin plans for implementation. Due to these factors, work to implement §3503 has not been initiated.

§4001 (National Prevention, Health Promotion, and Public Health Council) requires the President to establish an interagency National Prevention, Health Promotion, and Public Health Council. The Council must develop a strategy across Federal departments to prevent disease and promote the nation's health. The National Prevention Strategy was due by March 23, 2011. The National Prevention Strategy was published late on June 16, 2011, followed by the Annual Status Report which was made public on July 1, 2011.

§4108 (Medicaid Prevention and Wellness Incentives) requires the Secretary to award grants to states by January 1, 2011 for incentives to Medicaid beneficiaries who participate in evidence-based, healthy-lifestyle programs to prevent or help manage chronic disease. A report to Congress on these programs is due January 1, 2014. The availability of funds for the Medicaid Incentives for Prevention of Chronic Disease (MIPCD) program was announced in February 2011. On September 13, 2011, the following states were selected to receive grants: Wisconsin, Minnesota, New York, Nevada, New Hampshire, Montana, Hawaii, Texas, California, and Connecticut.

§4201 (Community Transformation Grants) requires the Secretary to establish a competitive grant program for the implementation, evaluation, and dissemination of evidence-based, community preventive health activities, focusing on prevalent chronic diseases such as diabetes and coronary artery disease. The program is being administered through the CDC in compliance with federal grant-making regulations. In FY2011, approximately $103 million in prevention funding was awarded to a total of 61 states and communities. Twenty-six states and communities will use awarded grants to build capacity for community prevention efforts. Thirty-five states and communities will use awarded grants to implement evidence- and practice-based programs designed to improve health and wellness.

§4202(a) (Community Wellness Pilot Program) requires the Secretary to award grants for a five-year pilot program to provide community prevention interventions, screenings, and clinical referrals for individuals aged 55 to 64. The ACA does not specify deadlines for establishment of the pilot program or the award of grants, and no funds for implementation have been identified. At a minimum, funding for staffing and evaluation of the project is necessary to begin plans for implementation.

§4202(b) (Medicare Prevention and Wellness Evaluation) requires the Secretary to conduct an evaluation of community-based prevention and wellness programs and, based on the findings, develop a plan to promote healthy lifestyles and chronic disease self-management among Medicare beneficiaries. A report to Congress on these matters is due by September 30, 2013. To date, no action has been taken on this provision.

§5604 (Co-Locating Primary and Specialty Care in Community-Based Mental Health Settings) requires the Secretary to fund demonstration projects for coordinated and integrated services to individuals with mental illness and co-occurring chronic diseases through the co-location of primary and specialty care services in community-based mental and behavioral health settings. There are no deadlines related to §5604 in the law, and no funds for implementation have been identified. At a minimum, funding for staffing and evaluation of the project is necessary to begin plans for implementation.

§10333 (Community-Based Collaborative Care Network Program) authorizes the Secretary to award grants to support "community-based collaborative care networks" in which comprehensive, coordinated, and integrated health care is provided to low-income populations. Grant funding may be used to perform health outreach, provide case management to low-income populations, and expand capacity through telehealth, after-hours services, or urgent care, among other uses. The ACA does not specify deadlines for §10333, and no grants have been awarded. To date, no funds for imple-

mentation have been identified, and work on the demonstrations has not been initiated.

In summary, primary and preventive care initiatives represent an important focus of new resources and efforts established by the ACA. Of the 14 tasks in this category, the Administration has implemented seven provisions, one provision has not hit its deadline, and one task (§3503) has not been appropriated and is past its deadline. Five provisions in this section did not have deadlines specified by law and did not have funding appropriated to them. To date, implementation of these five provisions has not yet begun.

Priority Area 3: Quality Measurement and Reporting

Quality measurement and reporting are prerequisites for implementing payment reform and mobilizing informed consumers as a force for change in health care. Payers and consumers will benefit from federal investments in quality measures development and deployment to improve the transparency of quality and value in the health care system. We identified ten provisions of the ACA concerned with quality measurement and reporting, including:

1. Medicaid Adult Health Quality Measures (§2701);
2. Quality Measures Reporting System for Long-Term Care Facilities (§3004);
3. Quality Reporting for Cancer Hospitals (§3005);
4. National Strategy for Health Care Quality (§3011);
5. Interagency Working Group on Health Care Quality (§3012);
6. Quality Measure Development; Development of Outcome Measures (§3013) (§10303);
7. Quality Measurement (§3014);
8. Data Collection; Public Reporting (§3015) (§10305);
9. Patient-Centered Outcomes Research (§6301); and
10. Quality Reporting for Psychiatric Hospitals (§10322).

Six of the ten quality measurement and reporting provisions have been implemented, one is partially complete, one provision does not have deadlines specified by law; and two provisions have deadlines in coming years.

§2701 (Medicaid Adult Health Quality Measures) requires the Secretary to identify and publish for comment recommended adult health quality measures for voluntary use by State Medicaid programs not later than January 1, 2011. The Secretary is also required, not later than January 1, 2012, to publish the initial core set of adult health quality measures applicable to Medicaid-eligible adults. The Secretary has met both of these deadlines: on December 30, 2010, the Secretary published a notice with comment period regarding recommended adult health quality measures; and on December 30, 2011, the Secretary released the initial core set of quality measures.

§3004 (Quality Measures Reporting System for Long-Term Care Facilities) would require long-term care hospitals, inpatient rehabilitation hospitals, and hospice programs to submit quality measure data starting in 2014 and for each subsequent year. If these facilities do not submit quality data, they will face a two-percent reduction in their annual update, increase factor for payments, or market basket percentage respectively. Not later than October 1, 2012, the Secretary must publish the quality measures selected for all three facility types that will be subject to reporting in 2014. The Secretary is required to report these quality measures on CMS' website. On August 4, 2011, the rules that specified the quality measures to be reported by hospices and inpatient rehabilitation facilities were published in the Federal Register. Shortly following, on August 18, 2011, the rule for long-term care facilities was published in the Federal Register as part of the final rules for "Hospital Inpatient Prospective Payment Systems for Acute Care Hospitals" and "Long-Term Care Hospital Prospective Payment System and FY 2012 Rates."

§3005 (Quality Reporting for Cancer Hospitals) would require cancer hospitals to submit quality data starting in FY2014 and for each subsequent fiscal year. By October 1, 2012, the Secretary must publish the quality measures selected for reporting in 2014. The Secretary is also required to report the quality measures that related to cancer hospitals on CMS' website. The Administration is working on a rule regarding quality measures for cancer hospitals, but it has not yet been published.

§3011 (National Strategy for Health Care Quality) requires the Secretary to establish and submit to Congress a national strategy to improve the delivery of health care services, patient health outcomes, and population health not later than January 1, 2011. The report is expected to be updated annually. The ACA also requires the Secretary to create a website with the following information by January 1, 2011: (1) national priorities for health care quality improvement; (2) agency-specific strategic plans for health care quality; and (3) other information, as the Secretary determines to be appropriate. On March 21, 2011, HHS released the national strategy titled, "Report to Congress: National Strategy for Quality Improvement in Health Care." AHRQ has created a webpage called "Working for Quality," found at www.ahrq. gov/workingforquality/about, which includes information about the National Quality Strategy, but does not include information about the agency-specific strategic plans.

§3012 (Interagency Working Group on Health Care Quality) establishes the Interagency Working Group on Health Care Quality, convened by the President and chaired by the Secretary, to submit to Congress and publish on the Internet, a report on its progress and recommendations. The initial report was due to Congress by December 31, 2010. The first annual report was sent to Congress on March 21, 2011.

HHS is in the process of developing the second annual report to Congress.

§3013 (Quality Measure Development) as amended by §10303 (Development of Outcome Measures) requires the Secretary, in consultation with AHRQ and CMS, to (1) identify, not less than triennially, gaps where no quality measures exist or where existing measures need improvement, updating, or expansion consistent with the National Strategy for Quality Improvement; and (2) award grants or contracts with eligible entities for the development, improvement, or expansion of quality measures. The initial set of measures should be made public by March 23, 2012. §10303 requires the Secretary to develop provider-level outcomes measures for hospital and physicians and outcome measures for acute and chronic disease and primary and preventive care. The law requires that for both acute and chronic disease and primary and preventive care not less than 10 outcome measures be developed 24 months after the date of enactment (March 23, 2012) and 36 months after the date of enactment (March 23, 2013), respectively. To meet its statutory requirements under §10303, HHS requested an expedited review by the National Quality Forum of readmissions measures. To date, HHS has not released provider-level outcomes measures for acute and chronic disease or primary and preventive care.

§3014 (Quality Measurement) expands the duties of the entity under contract with CMS pursuant to SSA §1890 (currently the National Quality Forum (NQF)). The ACA requires the entity to convene multi-stakeholder groups to provide input on national priorities for health care quality improvement (developed under the ACA). The stakeholder groups are also expected to weigh in on the selection of quality and efficiency measures for Medicare payment systems and other health care programs. This section establishes a multi-step pre-rulemaking process and timeline for the adoption, dissemination, and review of measures by the Secretary. The initial list of measures was published by the Secretary on December 2, 2011. The NQF is serving as the convener of the multi-stakeholder groups defined in this section, and has established the Measure Applications Partnership (MAP) to carry out its convening duties. As required by statute, a list of measures under consideration for 2012 rulemaking has been posted on NQF's website. MAP provided a report to HHS, based on this list of measures, recommending measures for inclusion in quality programs on February 1, 2012.

§3015 (Data Collection; Public Reporting) as amended by §10305 (Quality Measurement) requires the Secretary to collect and aggregate consistent data on quality and resource use measures from information systems used to support health care delivery to implement the public reporting of performance information, and may award grants or contracts for these purposes. The law also requires the Secretary to make available on the Internet performance information on quality measures. Section 10305 requires the Secretary to establish and implement a strategic framework to carry out the public reporting of performance information, including timelines for implementing nationally-consistent data collection, data aggregation, and analysis methods. There are no deadlines stipulated under §3015 or §10305.

§6301 (Patient-Centered Outcomes Research) establishes a private, nonprofit entity – the Patient-Centered Outcomes Research Institute (PCORI) – governed by a public-private sector board appointed by the Comptroller General to support and identify priorities for comparative effectiveness research. PCORI was established in September 2010, and issued its first call for pilot projects in the fall of 2011. There were 856 grant applications submitted for the first call, of which a total of 40 pilots will be funded.

§10322 (Quality Reporting for Psychiatric Hospitals) would require psychiatric hospitals and psychiatric units to submit quality data to the Secretary beginning in 2014 and for each subsequent year. Failure to report this data will result in a two percentage point reduction in a facilities' annual update to their federal rate for discharges. Not later than October 1, 2012, the Secretary is required to publish the quality measures selected for reporting by psychiatric hospitals in 2014. The Secretary is also required to publish the quality measures by posting them on CMS' website. CMS intends to propose quality measures and reporting requirements through rulemaking prior to the October 1, 2012 statutory deadline. The agency is currently seeking input from the psychiatric community, and held two "listening sessions" with stakeholders in 2011 to discuss the psychiatric facility quality reporting requirements of §10322 and the psychiatric measures that the agency is considering.[1]

The Administration has begun implementation on six provisions in this category (although the implementation of two tasks occurred after their statutory deadlines). Of the remaining four provisions, one is partially complete, two have not yet been implemented but are not past their deadlines, and one has not been implemented but does not have any statutorily-defined deadlines.

Priority Area 4: Administrative Simplification

We identified three ACA policies that promote administration simplification:

1. HIPAA Electronic Transactions Standards; Development of Standards for Administrative and Financial Transactions (§1104) (§10109);
2. Eligibility and Enrollment Systems (§1413); and
3. Standardized Complaint Form (§6105).

Two of the three provisions have deadlines and these policies have been implemented. The Administration has also taken action on the third provision, which does not have

statutorily-defined deadlines. This last provision is tied to the coverage portions of the ACA that take effect in 2014.

§1104 as amended by §10109 (HIPAA Electronic Transactions Standards) establishes a timeline, with multiple deadlines through January 1, 2016, for the Secretary to adopt and implement a single set of operating rules for each HIPAA administrative and financial electronic transaction for which there is an existing standard. The law establishes penalty fees, beginning in 2014, for health plans that fail to certify that their data systems comply with the most current HIPAA standards and associated operating rules. On July 8, 2011, HHS published an interim final rule adopting operating rules for health care claims status and health plan eligibility transactions. On January 5, 2012, HHS announced the interim final rule regarding new standards for electronic funds transfers. §10109 requires the Secretary, no later than January 1, 2012 and not less than every three years thereafter, to solicit input on whether there could be greater uniformity in financial and administrative activities from the National Committee on Vital and Health Statistics, the Health Information Technology Policy Committee, the Health Information Technology Standards Committee, and standard setting organizations and stakeholders.

§1413 (Eligibility and Enrollment Systems) requires the Secretary to establish a system in which residents of each state can apply for enrollment, receive a determination of eligibility, and continue participation in state health subsidy programs. The system must ensure that if an individual applying for an exchange is found eligible for Medicaid or the Children's Health Insurance Program, then the individual is enrolled for assistance under those programs. HHS released a final rule that implements the systems included in §1413 on March 12, 2012.

§6105 (Standardized Complaint Form) requires the Secretary to develop and make available a standardized complaint form to be used by residents (or their representatives) in filing complaints against a skilled nursing facility or a nursing facility. CMS posted a standardized complaint form and links to state complaint websites in updates to the Medicare Nursing Home Compare website on April 23, 2011.

In summary, the Administration has implemented or begun implementation of the three administrative simplification tasks reviewed in this section.

Priority Area 5: Health Information Technology

Three provisions of the ACA specifically target the adoption and effective use of health information technology (HIT):

1. Enrollment Standards (§1561);
2. Culture Change and Information Technology Demonstration Program (§6114); and
3. CMS Computer System Modernization (§10330).

Two of the three provisions have been implemented; the third provision, a demonstration project, has not been funded and is past its deadline.

§1561(Enrollment Standards) requires the Secretary, in consultation with the Health Information Technology (HIT) Policy Committee and the HIT Standards Committee, to develop interoperable and secure standards and protocols that facilitate enrollment of individuals in federal and state health and human services programs. The proposed standards and protocols were due by September 19, 2010. In August 2010, the HIT Policy and Standards Committees approved initial recommendations for a minimum set of standards and data elements. On September 17, 2010, the Secretary adopted these recommendations.

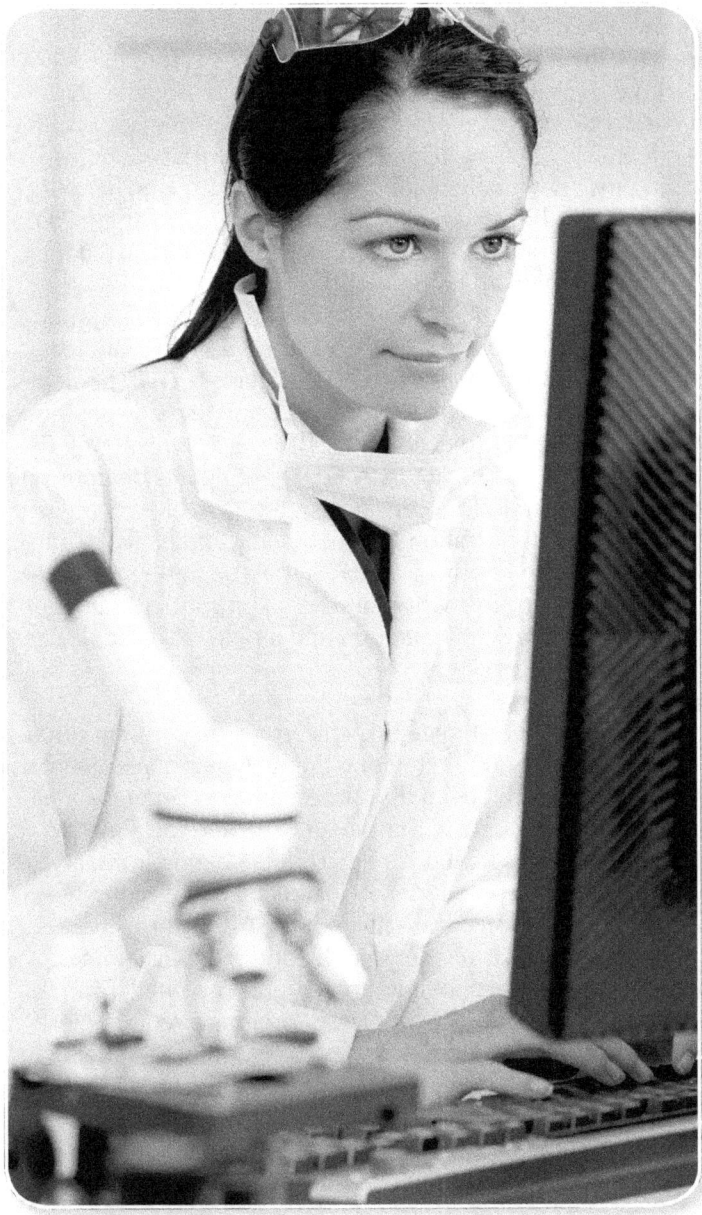

§6114 (Culture Change and Information Technology Demonstration Program) requires the Secretary, within one year of enactment (by March 23, 2011), to award one or more competitive grants to support each of the two following three-year demonstration projects for skilled nursing facilities and nursing facilities: (1) develop best practices for culture change (i.e., patient-centric models of care); and (2) develop best practices for the use of health information technology. The project does not include appropriation of implementation funding specific to it and no funds for implementation have been identified.

§10330 (CMS Computer System Modernization) requires the Secretary to develop and post a plan to modernize CMS' computer and data systems to support improvements in care delivery. The plan, which was due December 23, 2010, was expected to include a detailed budget for the resources needed for its implementation. On December 23, 2010, CMS released a report on its IT modernization program titled, "Modernizing CMS Computer and Data Systems to Support Improvements in Care Delivery, Version 1.0."

In summary, two of the three HIT-related policies introduced through the ACA have been implemented, and the third provision, the demonstration program, has not been appropriated for and has not been implemented on time.

Conclusion

In less than two years since the ACA was signed into law, most of the policies intended to promote delivery system reform have been implemented. The Administration has implemented 25 of 45 delivery system provisions fully, and has partially completed the implementation of two others. Of those that remain, six do not have deadlines, six are not yet due, and six are past their deadlines. Of the six provisions that are past deadlines, four are demonstration projects that have not received funding, one is a grant program that has not received funding, and one is a report to Congress.

The Administration's progress on the provisions reviewed in this chapter must be considered in light of the complexity and sheer number of reforms included in the Affordable Care Act, and strong resistance by some in Congress to the implementation and funding of the ACA. In the next chapter, we'll discuss the broad themes of implementation, remaining challenges, and opportunities to move health care delivery system reform forward.

ENDNOTES

1 Centers for Medicaid & Medicare Services. Affordable Care Act Section 10322 inpatient psychiatric hospital quality reporting listening session: Psychiatric measures under consideration. Retrieved from https://www.cms.gov/HospitalQualityInits/Downloads/HospitalPsychiatricMeasuresUnderConsideration.pdf

CHAPTER FIVE

Assessing Implementation and Looking Forward

"There are people right now who want to cut benefits and ration care and have that be the avenue to cost reduction in this country and that's wrong. It's so wrong, it's almost criminal. It's an inept way of thinking about health care."

George Halvorson, 2011[1]

The success of the Affordable Care Act (ACA) is critical to improving the sustainability of the U.S. health care system and the efficiency of care delivery. For the first time, because of the ACA, policymakers have the tools to focus on quality rather than quantity, efficiency rather than volume, and patients rather than their bottom line. These reforms also promise to deliver much-needed savings, and to do so in the most patient-centered way – by improving the quality of care and health outcomes. Steps must be taken to ensure the rapid and purposeful implementation of the law.

Unfortunately, since the ACA was signed into law, efforts have been made - on both federal and state levels - to dismantle federal health care programs and de-fund the law. For example, the Attorneys General of 26 states have pursued litigation that would invalidate the ACA. In the House of Representatives, one of the first pieces of legislation passed in the 112th Congress, H.R. 2, was to repeal the entire law. Some have proposed turning Medicare into a voucher program, or putting strict caps on Medicaid spending. These approaches to "reform" would greatly increase costs and out-of-pocket expenses for the 50 million American seniors and individuals with disabilities[2] and 69 million children and adults[3] who rely on Medicare and Medicaid, respectively. Describing these tactics, George Halvorson, the CEO of Kaiser Permanente, said, "It's an inept way of thinking about health care."[4] Not only do these proposals unfairly shift costs on seniors and low-income Americans, but they fail to deal with the underlying need for system-wide reform to address these costs in the first place.

In order to achieve meaningful and humane cost savings in the health care system, we must reengineer how care is delivered. Thankfully, there is a growing movement throughout the health care industry to prioritize and invest in reforming the health care delivery system. This movement – of doctors, hospitals, insurers, employers, and even some states – is driving innovation in care delivery to improve the quality, safety, and effectiveness of care. These innovating health care stakeholders are proving that changes to the way care is delivered result in significant improvements in cost and quality; not just in theory, but in practice.

To achieve the promise of increased efficiency and improved care, the federal government needs to promote innovative approaches to health care delivery that enable patients to receive the right care at the right time. The Affordable Care Act has these tools. Indeed, in reference to the delivery system reform provisions of the ACA, MIT Professor Jonathan Gruber said, "I can't think of a thing to try that [Congress] didn't try. They really made the best effort anyone has ever made. Everything is in here... I can't think of anything I'd do that they are not doing in the bill. You couldn't have done better than they are doing."[5]

Earlier in this report, we described the pressure of increasing health care costs in the U.S. The share of GDP dedicated to health care has tripled since 1960, and federal spending on health care is projected to rise from 5.5 percent of GDP now to about 14 percent in 2060. These figures demonstrate the urgent need for delivery system reform. A key challenge facing the Administration is how quickly and effectively the delivery system reforms in the ACA can be implemented and expanded upon. This will require a significant coordination effort across the Administration and a plan for reshaping our health care system.

We do not underestimate this challenge, particularly since responsibility for implementing the ACA cuts across federal departments and federal and state agencies. Federal agencies must coordinate with state, county, and local governments, as well as health care providers ranging from large hospitals to solo practitioners, insurers, and community-based organizations. The Office of the Inspector General (OIG) at the Department of Health and Human Services described the oversight and implementation challenges that HHS faces in this way: "Many programs require close coordination between the Department and other federal and state agencies. Additional ongoing implementation and operational challenges include the magnitude, complexity, and novelty of programs; compressed implementation timelines; and marketplace dynamics."[6]

As the OIG notes, the cross-cutting nature of the ACA's

reforms makes communication and coordination across the federal government and existing health care delivery systems a critical component of the implementation process. For example, the Medicare Shared Savings Program (§3022) involved the coordination of rulemaking within various parts of HHS, the Federal Trade Commission, the Department of Justice, and the Internal Revenue Service. Managing the timing and coordination of programs, like §3022, that require action from several federal agencies will be an ongoing implementation challenge for the Administration. Of course, even the most coordinated federal effort will face the challenge of reforming a disorganized, fragmented health care system that for years has reinforced the wrong incentives; incentives that place a priority on quantity rather than quality of care.

This reform will need to disentangle existing systems and the perverse patterns of behavior in our current health care system. For example, before the ACA, Medicare payment policy did little to incent acute-care providers to coordinate patients' transition to non-acute care settings. The ACA introduces reforms that change incentive structures to better align hospital payments to patient outcomes. **CMS estimates that payment adjustment, among other reforms, will result in a 20 percent reduction in hospital readmission rates by 2013.** However, stakeholders who are invested in the status quo will present a challenge to the Administration as it works on restructuring the delivery of care to address misaligned incentives, inefficient systems, and incongruous behavior.

In spite of these challenges, the Obama Administration already has made significant progress implementing the delivery system provisions of the Affordable Care Act. In the previous chapter, we found that of the 45 delivery system reform provisions in the ACA, 25 have been implemented in accordance with statutory deadlines. Of the 20 reforms that remain, six provisions do not have deadlines associated with them, six provisions are not yet due, two provisions are partially complete, and six provisions have not received funding and were not implemented in accordance with statutory deadlines.

It is important that the Administration continue to prioritize delivery system reform. To this end, the Administration must develop a strategy for how to coordinate, sequence, and communicate the implementation of each reform. In this chapter, we assess the Administration's implementation efforts, focusing on whether the organization of implementation has been coordinated across federal agencies, appropriately sequenced, and adheres to coherent themes.

Coordination

Coordination is key to successful implementation of any complex reform. In this context, effective coordination

begins with a concerted effort to manage implementation activities horizontally within HHS and across federal agencies. The coordination also must be vertical, from the federal level to state, local, and community-based providers. The Administration uses the law's requirements and deadlines as the starting point for implementation plans. Each provision of the law is assigned a primary "home" within HHS. The "home" agency or office is responsible for making the provision operational and developing detailed project and implementation plans. These plans then guide the decision- and priority-making processes as implementation moves forward.

The ACA requires the Secretary to consult and coordinate implementation with several federal agencies within the HHS, and also other federal departments, state governments, and health care stakeholders. For example, as part of developing quality and efficiency measures (§3013), the Secretary must consult with the Director of the Agency for Healthcare Research and Quality and the Administrator of the Centers for Medicaid & Medicare Services. For the grant program authorized under §3503, the Secretary is required to work with a broad spectrum of entities, including federal, state, private, public-private, health care organizations, consumer advocates, chronic disease groups, and other stakeholders, to design medication therapy management services.

In instances when programs overlap, or one provision requires the oversight and expertise of multiple agencies, the Office of the Secretary coordinates an inter-agency process in which working groups and policy teams are created from representatives of each agency. Senior managers are responsible for resolving how programs are constructed to achieve their policy goal, and how to coordinate efforts to ensure a consistent implementation timeline across agencies. Coordination of efforts also is facilitated by the White House Office of Health Reform, which helps to set strategic priorities and ensure alignment across departments and agencies.

HHS has recognized that effective coordination will require more than just the statutory requirements of the ACA. For example, ongoing management of delivery system reform implementation will be aided by a new mechanism for tracking the success of health reform recently initiated by HHS. **The Assistant Secretary for Planning and Evaluation will soon launch a public, online health reform "dashboard" that will include data and trends on national health expenditures.** The dashboard is an opportunity to better understand, track, and evaluate how health care reform affects health care spending over time. This initiative, which is not required under the ACA, will be a useful tool to target spending trends in specific areas of the health industry. We encourage HHS to continue to develop initiatives like the health reform dashboard so that Congress and the general public can be more effectively engaged with the Administration's ongoing efforts.

Sequencing

In addition to coordination, it is important that the Administration is attentive to the sequence of implementing provisions of the ACA. We define sequencing as the logical and complementary ordering of reform efforts. For example, robust quality measures and widespread adoption of health IT facilitate providers' ability to measure and report quality information. The implementation of payment reforms, like the Medicare Shared Savings program, relies on providers' ability to measure and report quality information. Appropriately sequencing health care reforms could improve the efficiency with which the health care industry adapts to the new payment systems, reporting requirements, and new models of care delivery required by the ACA.

The Administration, in determining how to sequence implementation, takes into account statutory requirements, the policy history, existing programs, and developed technology that can contribute to informing the implementation of a provision. Obviously, meeting statutory deadlines are the Administration's first priority. Where the law directs that the Secretary shall implement X provision by Y date, the Administration acts according to the statutorily-defined sequence. As discussed in the previous chapter, the Administration has successfully met the majority of deadlines for delivery system reforms in the ACA.

Other provisions of the law, like the Center for Medicare and Medicaid Innovation (§3021), give discretion to the Secretary to identify priorities. In these instances, the Administration has taken advantage of preexisting infrastructure to accelerate certain reforms. For example, CMS collaborated with Premier, Inc. on a hospital pay-for-performance demonstration project between 2003 and 2009. Based on this prior work, the Hospital Value-Based Purchasing Program (§3001) moved forward quickly. Specifically, the pay-for-performance demonstration program developed the systems and infrastructure for hospital reporting of quality measurements which enabled the Administration to implement a robust value-based purchasing system for in-patient hospitals. In contrast, the Physician Value-Based Modifier (§3007), which will apply to all physicians in 2017, is an area where there is less programmatic precedent and infrastructure for CMS and health care providers to build from. The implementation of §3007 will involve more work by CMS and providers to ensure that the necessary technology and infrastructure is available.

Where the law gives discretion, there are opportunities for the Administration to sequence reforms to ensure the most effective and efficient implementation. Last year, the Innovation Center implemented a number of initiatives and care models, including the Partnership for Patients, the State Demonstrations to Integrate Care for Dual Eligible Individuals, the Innovation Advisors Program, Federally Qualified Health Centers Advanced Primary Care demonstration, and the CMS Health Care Innovation Challenge.[7] These programs go through rigorous, inter-departmental and inter-agency processes to ensure that the established goals and timelines are consistent with the Administration's priorities. As the Administration learns from the Innovation Center's work on these early models and demonstrations, other areas of research and innovation may be identified and prioritized to advance the aims of health reform.

In many respects, the Administration's sequencing of implementation is understandable: statutory requirements come first, and areas in which comparable reforms already have been piloted will advance more quickly. Going forward, we encourage the Administration to focus its efforts on the "building blocks" of reform; particularly, the information and payment system that are the basis of the daily interaction among patients, providers, and payers. We also encourage the Administration to focus its efforts on communicating these changes to providers through the health care systems, from large hospitals to solo practitioners. Long-term sustainability of reform efforts will require understanding and buy-in from those who provide health care services.

Themes

Organizing implementation of the ACA around meaningful policy themes, goals, and objectives is also important. With such a complex task at hand, simple, measurable themes help communicate goals and provide the basis for measuring success. The following overarching policy themes reach across the ACA's five priority areas of delivery system reform:

- Improving coordination of care across the care continuum;
- Enhancing prevention and addressing drivers of chronic disease;
- Promoting quality and value of care;
- Putting the needs of patients first; and
- Reducing overall health care costs.

Several provisions of the ACA fall under, but address different aspects of, the same theme. According to Administration officials, when programs touch upon similar themes, staffs collaborate on a project plan that identifies the common policy goals and direction. Particular attention is paid to understanding how provisions overlap and how implementation affects the incentive structures in the delivery system. For example, there are several provisions of the ACA's delivery system reforms that touch on the theme of improving coordination of care across the care continuum. Some of these reforms include the Hospital Readmission Reduction Program (§3025), National Pilot Program on Payment Bundling (§3023), the Community-Based Transitions Program (§3026), and the Independence at Home Demonstration Program (§3024). These provisions, which enact new payment incentives and penalties and test new models for post-acute and community-based care, contribute, in different ways, to achieving the same policy goal. The focus on overarching policy objectives, rather than individual policies, orients implementation towards approaches that can achieve the best outcomes.

The Administration has identified policy themes in the ACA, and coordinates reforms that touch upon similar themes. However, coordinating reforms along identified themes will not be sufficient to sustain the momentum of implementation. For each policy theme, the Administration should establish benchmarks, goals, and tracking systems. We have seen this, for example, with the Partnership for Patients initiative. This initiative's goal to reduce hospital readmissions by 20 percent over three years is tied to the theme of coordination of care across the care continuum. The Administration should undertake the exercise of setting benchmarks and goals within each of its identified policy themes.

Over time, having benchmarks and tracking systems will enable policymakers to better understand which programs are effective and should be prioritized for expansion. We urge the Administration, in setting benchmarks and tracking outcomes, to continue to be transparent in publicly displaying or otherwise communicating that information to the public, Congress, and states.

Looking Forward

Our debt and deficit, and the pressure from rising health care costs, should compel the U.S. toward health care delivery system reform. Businesses across the country have seen their bottom lines eroded by uncontrollable health care costs; would-be wage increases are consumed by increasing health care costs; and ordinary Americans find decent health insurance ever harder to afford. The advantage of addressing our health care cost problem through health care delivery system reform is that the benefits will accrue throughout the economy; not just to Medicare, but to businesses large and small, to states and municipalities, to workers and health care consumers.

In Chapter 3, we identified several examples of health care organizations that are realizing the potential of delivery system reform to transform our health care system. These case studies show that enormous improvement in our health care system is possible. **The U.S. health care system can change from one of the world's least efficient, most complicated, and most frustrating systems for patients and providers, to one that can be the envy of the world.**

The potential cost savings involved are enormous. As we've noted before, the President's Council of Economic Advisors estimated that over $700 billion a year can be saved without compromising health outcomes, the Institutes of Medicine put this number at $765 billion, the New England Healthcare Institute reported that it is $850 billion annually, and the Lewin Group and former Bush Treasury Secretary Paul O'Neill have estimated the savings at $1 trillion – each and every year.

In passing the ACA, Congress enacted a blueprint for how the health care delivery system will be reformed over the next several years, focusing on value, quality, and reducing overall per-capita costs. The Administration's ability to maintain momentum for delivery system reform will be a significant issue moving forward. The ongoing implementation of the ACA is a tremendous effort for the Administration, state leaders, and health care stakeholders. Ensuring that delivery system reform remains a priority across the health care industry and federal and State governments is a pressing challenge facing implementation.

To maintain the pace of implementation, we recommend that the Administration enhance its communication to stakeholders and set a cost-savings target for the law's delivery system reforms. Addressing these issues will facilitate the implementation of the ACA and encourage continued efforts toward delivery system reform.

Enhanced Communication

Payment reforms have been among the first of the ACA's delivery system reforms to be made operational since the bill was signed into law. However, the Administration's expectations regarding delivery system reform are not limited to payment reform. It expects health care providers to undertake and make progress on each of the five priority areas at once, with an eye toward reducing overall health care costs. This "all-fronts" approach to delivery system reform is difficult for health care providers to manage; not only for rural community providers, but also for advanced health care organizations like Geisinger Health System.

Regardless of the care setting, making new care delivery models work involves substantial risk, financial and otherwise, for health care providers. While some of the larger, integrated health care systems have the staff and infrastructure in place to undertake multiple reform projects at the same time, other providers are not prepared for the onslaught of new programs, payment systems, and regulations stemming from the ACA. For the providers that fall into the latter category, deciding which direction they should move in first can be confusing.

We recommend the Administration enhance its outreach and communications efforts to health care providers and clearly articulate its policy priorities for delivery system reform. The dashboard is a good start, and shows that there are actions the Secretary can take under her existing authority to move the ball forward. Providing the health care industry with additional guidance on which aspects of reform should take precedence will enable providers to target manpower and investments. A clear signal from the Administration about policy goals and how providers should prioritize delivery system reforms to reach those goals will help keep providers on the same page and moving in the same direction.

A Cost-Savings Target

In 1961, President Kennedy declared that within ten years the U.S. would put a man on the moon and return him safely. This message, and the mission outlined, was clear, direct, and accountable. The result was a vast mobilization of private and public resources that collaborated in innovative ways to achieve that purpose. While the issue facing our country is different, the urgency – and the need to mobilize public and private sectors toward improving quality and lowering costs in our health care system – is the same.

To this end, we encourage the Administration to set a cost-savings target for delivery system reform. A cost-savings target will focus, guide, and spur the Administration's efforts in a manner that vague intentions to "bend the health care cost curve" will not. It also would provide a measurable goal by which we can evaluate the progress of implementation.

In this report, we noted various experts' estimates on the savings that can be achieved through health care delivery system reform. If the President's Council of Economic Advisers' $700 billion savings estimate is correct, since Medicare amounts to 20 percent of America's health care spending, we could save $42 billion a year in Medicare cost if we only achieved 30 percent of the potential. Over a ten-year budget period, that's $420 billion in Medicare savings -- all without taking away any benefits, and while likely improving care.

Setting a goal will help overcome some of the roadblocks we face making this vision of our health care system a reality. When it comes to federal policy, for example, the legislative process places too significant a focus on short-term savings. Cost analyses of specific federal programs often undervalue or simply do not measure the possible effect of how changes in federal law will drive down the cost of providing health care in the private sector. As the Congressional Budget Office has acknowledged, "In some cases, estimating the budgetary effects of a proposal is hampered by limited evidence. Studies generally examine the effects of discrete policy changes but typically do not address what would happen if several changes were made at the same time. Those interactions could mean that the savings from combining two or more initiatives will be greater than or less than the sum of their individual effects."[8]

Now is the time for the Administration to set a clear challenge for itself, states, and private industry. Announcing an overarching goal for delivery system reform savings will drive forward progress, and generate momentum to achieve that goal. We urge the Administration to take action on this issue.

Given the complexity of our health care system and delivery system reform, the Administration has worked quickly to organize its internal processes and has successfully moved forward in all reform sectors and on most key provisions of the ACA. In this chapter, we described the Administration's internal processes to coordinate implementation efforts across federal agencies and found that the Administration conceptualizes the law along broad policy themes, like care coordination, prevention of chronic disease, promoting quality and value, and reducing health care costs. While the sequencing of implementation is largely dictated in the first instance by the law, where discretion is given to HHS, or in the out years as programs continue, we recommend the Administration pay more attention to how sequencing can improve efficiency, and enhance communication of policy priorities to health care providers.

Finally, we believe the implementation effort would benefit from a public announcement by the Administration identifying a savings target for health care delivery system reform and communicating a clear vision of the future to the public. Setting a hard challenge will raise the stakes and heighten the sense of urgency among the federal government, states, and private industry to seek, implement, and expand upon delivery system reform. With skyrocketing costs in our health care system at the heart of the U.S. budget deficit problem, we cannot wait to act on reducing costs and improving care in our health care system.

ENDNOTES

[1] Halvorson, G. (2011, September). Introduction at the Partnership for Quality Care Conference, Washington, DC. Retrieved from http://www.pqc-usa.org/pages?id=0003

[2] Davis, P. (2012, January). *Medicare primer*. (CRS report R40425). Washington, DC: Congressional Research Service.

[3] Herz, E. (2012). *Medicaid: A primer*. (CRS Report RL33202). Washington, DC: Congressional Research Service.

[4] Halvorson, G. (2011, September). Introduction at the Partnership for Quality Care Conference, Washington, DC. Retrieved from http://www.pqc-usa.org/pages?id=0003

[5] Brownstein, R. (2009, November 21). A milestone in the health care journey. *Atlantic*. Retrieved from http://www.theatlantic.com/politics/archive/2009/11/a-milestone-in-the-health-care-journey/30619/

[6] Office of the Inspector General, Department of Health and Human Services. *2011 Top management & performance challenge*. Retrieved from http://oig.hhs.gov/reports-and-publications/top-challenges/2011/

[7] Blum, J. (2011, November 10). *Responses to questions for the record at the Senate HELP Committee Hearing, "Improved Quality, Lower Costs: The Role of Health Care Delivery System Reform."* Washington, DC.

[8] Elmendorf, D. (2009, March 10). *Options for controlling the cost and increasing the efficiency of health care: Testimony before the House Subcommittee on Health, Committee of Energy and Commerce.* Washington, DC. Retrieved from http://cbo.gov/ftpdocs/100xx/doc10016/03-10-Health_Care.pdf

CHAPTER SIX

Conclusion

"Many of the specific changes that might ultimately prove most important cannot be foreseen today and could be developed only over time through experimentation and learning."

Doug Elmendorf, 2009[1]

The Administration's progress on the Affordable Care Act (ACA), and actions taken by key private-sector leaders, has put our health care system on the road to a more efficient delivery system. As we outline in Chapter 1, rising costs in the U.S. health care system compel the need for system-wide reform. In Chapter 2, we make the case that delivery system reform – particularly within the priority areas of payment reform, measuring and reporting quality, primary and preventive care, administrative simplification, and health information technology – holds the promise to significantly reduce costs while improving quality. Moreover, delivery system reform has the advantage of being a system-wide solution. It will improve the sustainability of Medicare, Medicaid, and TRICARE, and sharpen the competitive advantage of private-sector health care industries.

As we discuss, the private sector already recognizes that these investments control costs and improve care. Congress should learn from these lessons. In Chapter 3, we highlight the work of private-sector and local organizations that have already invested in delivery system reform, and are seeing results. Indeed, these organizations view the reforms they have made to their care delivery systems to be integral to building a sustainable business model. The exemplars described in Chapter 3 are evidence that significant reductions in health care costs can be achieved; not by taking away benefits, but by delivering better and more efficient care; a true win-win.

In the two years since the ACA was enacted, the Administration has made considerable progress implementing the law. In Chapter 4, we outline the status of 45 of the ACA's delivery system reforms, and find that the Administration has implemented 25 provisions fully and made progress on two others. The complexity and sheer number of reforms included the law make this accomplishment all the more noteworthy. In addition to the hurdles presented by our fragmented health care system, resistance by some in Congress to supporting the Administration's implementation efforts also creates barriers to swift implementation. For the 20 delivery system provisions that have not yet been implemented, we found that the lack of Congressional funding support is a significant factor in delaying forward progress.

We encourage members of Congress to fully fund the delivery system reform provisions that are outlined in this report. Failing to fund these provisions only serves to slow the rate at which we tackle the issue of controlling costs in our health care system – a goal on which stakeholders from all political persuasions agree. In many other ways the ACA is supporting and building upon the efforts undertaken by the private sector by realigning incentives in the health care system. A broad array of pilot and demonstration programs have been launched from which best practices will be deployed nationwide. The process to get to a more sustainable path will be one of "experimentation and learning," according to Doug Elmendorf, the Director of the Congressional Budget Office. The ACA creates the conditions that allow innovation to take place and has the mechanisms needed to propagate reforms as quickly as possible when they are proven effective. American ingenuity can overcome the toughest challenges, not through command and control but through dynamic, flexible, and persistent experimentation, learning, and encouragement. We need to trust that the path of innovation and experimentation is the right one, and not give up on these efforts.

When President Kennedy announced in September of 1962 that America would strive to put a man on the Moon, he said, "We choose to do such things not because they are easy, but because they are hard, because that goal will serve to organize and measure the best of our energies and skills, because that challenge is one that we are willing to accept, one we are unwilling to postpone, and one which we intend to win."[2]

We accept the challenge posed by the rising health care costs in our system, and know that we cannot postpone finding a solution. We can win this challenge, and drive our system toward a sustainable path of higher-quality care and improved outcomes, by supporting the Affordable Care Act.

ENDNOTES

[1] Elmendorf, Douglas. (2009, June 16). Letter to the Honorable Kent Conrad. Washington, D.C.: Congressional Budget Office. Retrieved from http://www.cbo.gov/sites/default/files/cbofiles/ftpdocs/103xx/doc10311/06-16-healthreformandfederalbudget.pdf

[2] Kennedy, J. (1962, September). Address at Rice University on the nation's space effort. Houston, TX. Retrieved from http://www.jfklibrary.org/Research/Ready-Reference/JFK-Speeches/Address-at-Rice-University-on-the-Nations-Space-Effort-September-12-1962.aspx

Appendix A

Geisinger 40 Best Practices for CABG Surgery

1. Preadmission documentation:

a. ACC/AHA indication
b. Screening for and consultation re: IMI/RV involvement
c. Treatment options and patient preference
d. Need for warfarin (anterior MI or wall motion abnormality)
e. Current user of clopidogrel or warfarin?
f. Screening for stroke risk
g. Carotid doppler (if the test is indicated)
h. Vascular surgery consultation (if indicated)
i. Ejection fraction
j. Screening for need to use intra-aortic balloon pump (IABP)
k. Screening using epiaortic echo (as indicated)
l. Patient withheld clopidogrel/warfarin for 5 d preoperatively?

2. Operative documentation:

a. Patient received correct dosing of beta-blocker (preoperative)
b. Correct use of intra-aortic balloon pump (preoperative 3 postoperative)
c. Preoperative antibiotic (within 60 min of incision; Vancomycin within 120 min)
d. Blood cardioplegia (on-pump patients)
e. Epiaortic echo of the ascending aorta and the peer consult
f. Intraoperative hyperglycemia screening
g. Correct insulin management (as indicated; per protocol)
h. Use of LIMA for LAD grafting

3. Postoperative patient documentation:

a. Anteroapical MI within prior 7 d: postoperative echo
b. Monitoring for atrial fibrillation for _48 h
c. Anticoagulation therapy (as indicated)
d. Antibiotic administered (postoperative for 24–48 h)
e. Aspirin (6 hours postoperative or 24 h postoperative)
f. Beta-blocker (within 24 h postoperative)
g. Statin administered (postoperative)
h. Surgical debridement and revascularization of any sternal wound infection
i. Plastic surgery consult regarding ongoing management of sterna wound
j. Tobacco screening and counseling

4. Discharge documentation:

a. Referral to cardiac rehabilitation
b. Discharge medications (eg, beta-blocker)
c. Discharge medication: aspirin
d. Discharge medication: statin

5. Post-Discharge documentation:

a. Patient correctly taking beta-blocker?
b. Patient correctly taking aspirin?
c. Patient correctly taking statin?
d. Patient correctly administering anticoagulant?
e. Did patient resume smoking?
f. Patient enrolled in cardiac rehabilitation?

Appendix B

Affordable Care Act Delivery System Reform Status Chart

ACA Section	Summary of Provision	Selected Deadlines	Implementation Actions Taken
PAYMENT REFORM			
2702	**Medicaid Payment Adjustment for Health Care-Acquired Conditions.** Requires the Secretary to promulgate regulations specifying health care-acquired conditions for which Medicaid payment is prohibited.	Regulations to take effect by July 1, 2011.	On June 6, 2011, CMS published a final rule prohibiting Medicaid payment for certain specified health care-acquired conditions (76 Federal Register 32816). CMS will delay compliance actions until July 1, 2012.
2704	**Medicaid Bundled Payment Demonstration.** Establishes a five-year demonstration project (Jan. 1, 2012 through Dec. 31, 2016), in up to eight states, to study the use of bundled payments for hospital and physician services under Medicaid.	Establish a demo project by Jan. 1, 2012. Report to Congress due one year after conclusion of demonstration project.	This provision has not received the funding needed to commence implementation.
2705	**Medicaid Global Payment System Demonstration Project.** Establishes a demonstration project for FY2010 through 2012 under which up to five states would adjust their Medicaid payment models for eligible safety-net hospital systems or networks.	Establish a demo project in FY2010. Report to Congress due one year after completion.	This provision has not received the funding needed to commence implementation.
2706	**Medicaid Pediatric Accountable Care Organization Demonstration Program.** Requires the Secretary to conduct a five-year demonstration project (Jan. 1, 2012 through Dec. 31, 2016), under which a participating state is allowed to recognize pediatric providers as an accountable care organization (ACO) for the purpose of receiving incentive payments. Authorizes the appropriation of such sums as may be necessary (SSAN) for the project.	Establish a demo program by Jan. 1, 2012.	This provision has not received the funding needed to commence implementation.
2707	**Medicaid Emergency Psychiatric Demonstration Project.** Establishes a three-year demonstration project for states to provide payment to "institutions for mental disease" for providing medical assistance for Medicaid-eligible individuals ages 21-65 who require medical attention for an emergency medical condition.	Report to Congress by Dec. 31, 2013 evaluating the demo project's affect on access to care and cost.	On March 13, 2012, CMS announced that 11 States and the District of Columbia have been selected to participate in the demonstration, including Alabama, California, Connecticut, Illinois, Maine, Maryland, Missouri, North Carolina, Rhode Island, Washington, and West Virginia.
3001(a)	**Hospital Value-Based Purchasing Program.** Establishes a value-based purchasing (VBP) program for hospitals starting in FY2013, under which value-based incentive payments will be made based on hospital performance on quality measures related to common and high-cost conditions such as cardiac, surgical, and pneumonia care. The hospital VBP program does not include measures of hospital readmissions.	Value-based incentive payments are for hospital discharges on or after Oct. 1, 2012.	CMS's final rule to implement the hospital VBP program was published on May 6, 2011 (76 Federal Register 26490). Note: the final rule updating Medicare inpatient hospital payment policies and rates for FY2012 (due to be published in the Federal Register on Aug. 18, 2011) adopts a Medicare spending per beneficiary measure for the new hospital VBP program, as required by ACA. On November 1, 2011, CMS released its final rule on the FY2014 VBP program.

ACA Section	Summary of Provision	Selected Deadlines	Implementation Actions Taken
3001(b)	**Value-Based Purchasing Demonstration Program.** Establishes two 3-year VBP demonstration programs for: (1) inpatient critical access hospitals; and (2) hospitals excluded from the VBP program due to insufficient number of measures and cases. The Secretary must report to Congress no later than 18 months after the completion of the demonstration programs.	The demo programs must be est. by March 23, 2013. Report to Congress 18 months after completion.	This provision has not received the funding needed to commence implementation.
3006; 10301	**Value-Based Purchasing Programs for Skilled Nursing Facilities, Home Health Agencies, and Ambulatory Surgical Centers.** Requires the Secretary to develop a plan to implement a Medicare VBP program for SNFs, home health agencies, and ambulatory surgical centers (ASC).	Report to Congress including the plan for a VBP program for SNFs and HH was due Oct. 1, 2011. A plan for ASC was due Jan. 1, 2011.	CMS released reports to Congress on the VBP implementation plan for ambulatory surgical centers and home health agencies. The VBP plan for ASC can be found at https://www.cms.gov/ASCPayment/downloads/C_ASC_RTC%202011.pdf. The home health VBP plan can be found at https://www.cms.gov/center/hha.asp. The report for skilled nursing facilities has not yet been released. It is in the process of final review within the Administration.
3007	**Physician Value-Based Payment Modifier.** Requires the Secretary to develop and implement a budget-neutral payment system that will adjust Medicare physician payments based on the quality and cost of the care they deliver. Quality and cost measures will be risk-adjusted and geographically standardized. The new payment system is to be phased in over a two-year period beginning in 2015.	Payment adjustments apply to certain physicians beginning on Jan. 1, 2015, and apply to all physicians by Jan. 1, 2017.	Quality of care and cost measures for the value-based payment modifier were included in CMS's final rule updating Medicare payment policies and rates for physician services paid under the Physician Fee Schedule in CY2012, which was published on Nov. 28, 2011 (76 *Federal Register* 73026). Under the rule, CY2013 is the initial performance year for purposes of adjusting payments in CY2015. For more information, see CMS fact sheet dated Nov. 1, 2011, at http://www.cms.gov/apps/media/fact_sheets.asp.
3008	**Hospital-Acquired Condition Payment Adjustment.** Starting in FY2015, hospitals in the top 25th percentile of rates of hospital-acquired conditions (HACs) for certain high-cost and common conditions will be subject to a payment penalty under Medicare. Requires the Secretary to report to Congress on the appropriateness of establishing a health care-acquired condition policy related to other providers participating in Medicare, including nursing homes, inpatient rehabilitation facilities, long-term care hospitals, outpatient hospital departments, ambulatory surgical centers, and health clinics.	Report to Congress due by Jan. 1, 2012; payment adjustments are for hospital discharges on or after Oct. 1, 2014.	The report to Congress on expanding HAC penalties to non-hospital providers has not yet been released. It is undergoing final review within the Administration.

ACA Section	Summary of Provision	Selected Deadlines	Implementation Actions Taken
3021	**Center for Medicare and Medicaid Innovation (CMMI).** Requires the Secretary, no later than Jan. 1, 2011, to establish the CMMI within CMS. The purpose of CMMI is to test and evaluate innovative payment and service delivery models to reduce program expenditures under Medicare, Medicaid, and CHIP while preserving or enhancing the quality of care furnished under these programs. Appropriates $5 million for FY2010 for the selection, testing, and evaluation of new payment and service delivery models; and $10 billion for the period FY2011 through FY2019, plus $10 billion for each subsequent 10-fiscal year period, to continue such activities and for the expansion and nationwide implementation of successful models.	Effective Jan. 1, 2011.	CMMI has 13 initiatives and demonstrations underway: • Advance Payment ACO Model. • Pioneer ACO Model (see Dec. 19, 2011 announcement at http://www.hhs.gov/news/press/2011pres/12/20111219a.html). • Bundled Payments for Care Improvement: testing four bundled payment models for services received during a defined episode of care. • Comprehensive Primary Care Initiative: working with commercial and state health insurance plans to offer bonus payments to primary care doctors who better coordinate patient care. • FQHC Advanced Primary Care Practice Demonstration: paying FQHCs a monthly care management fee to coordinate care for Medicare beneficiaries. • Health Care Innovation Challenge: grants to identify and test innovative care delivery and payment models. • Innovation Advisors Program: creating a network of experts in improving the delivery of care under Medicare, Medicaid, and CHIP. • Partnership for Patients: a national initiative aimed at reducing hospital-acquired conditions by 40% and hospital readmissions by 20% by the end of 2013. • State Demonstrations to Integrate Care for Dual Eligible Individuals: contracting with states to coordinate care for dual eligibles. • Financial Models to Support State Efforts to Integrate Care for Medicare and Medicaid Beneficiaries. • Initiative to Reduce Avoidable Hospitalizations among Nursing Facility Residents. • Million Hearts • Strong Start for Mothers and Newborns For more information on each of CMI's programs and activities, see http://innovations.cms.gov/.
3022	**Medicare Shared Savings Program.** Directs the Secretary to implement an integrated care delivery model using Accountable Care Organizations (ACOs), modeled on integrated delivery systems. While ACOs can be designed with varying features, most models put primary care physicians at the core, along with other providers, and emphasize simultaneously reducing costs and improving quality. Under the Medicare Shared Savings Program, CMS will contract for ACOs to assume responsibility for improving quality of care provided, coordinating care across providers, and reducing the cost of care Medicare beneficiaries receive. If cost and quality targets are met, ACOs will receive a share of any savings realized by CMS.	Effective Jan. 1, 2012.	CMS's final rule to implement the Medicare shared savings program was published on Nov. 2, 2011 (76 *Federal Register* 67802). Three additional documents have been issued in connection with the shared savings program final rule: (1) a joint CMS and HHS/OIG interim final rule with comment period establishing waivers of the application of the physician self-referral (Stark) law and the federal anti-kickback statute to ACOs (76 Federal Register 67992; Nov. 2, 2011); (2) a joint FTC and DOJ final policy statement regarding the application of federal antitrust laws to ACOs (76 Federal Register 67026; Oct. 28, 2011); and (3) an IRS notice summarizing how existing IRS guidance may apply to tax-exempt organizations such as charitable hospitals that participate in ACOs (IRS Notice 2011-20; Apr. 18, 2011).

ACA Section	Summary of Provision	Selected Deadlines	Implementation Actions Taken
3023	**National Medicare Payment Bundling Pilot Program.** Requires the Secretary to establish a five-year national, voluntary pilot program encouraging hospitals, doctors, and post-acute care providers to improve patient care and achieve savings for the Medicare program through bundled payment models. Before Jan. 1, 2016, the Secretary is also required to submit a plan to Congress to expand the pilot program if doing so will improve patient care and reduce spending. Authorizes the Secretary to expand the pilot program if it is found to improve quality and reduce costs. Also, directs the Secretary to test bundled payment arrangements involving continuing care hospitals within the bundling pilot program.	Pilot to be established by Jan. 1, 2013.	This provision has not received the funding needed to commence implementation.
3025	**Hospital Readmissions Reduction Program.** Beginning in FY2013, adjusts payments for hospitals paid under the inpatient prospective payment system based on the dollar value of each hospital's percentage of potentially preventable Medicare readmissions for the three conditions with risk-adjusted readmission measures that are currently endorsed by the NQF (i.e., acute myocardial infarction (heart attack), heart failure, and pneumonia). Authorizes the Secretary to expand the policy to additional conditions in future years and directs the Secretary to calculate and make publicly available information on all hospital patient readmission rates for certain conditions.	Payment reductions are for hospital discharges on or after Oct. 1, 2012.	CMS's final rule updating Medicare inpatient hospital payment policies and rates for FY2012, which was published on Aug. 18, 2011 (76 *Federal Register* 51476), finalizes readmissions measures and the methodology that will be used to calculate excess readmission rates. For more information, see CMS fact sheet dated Aug. 1, 2011, at http://www.cms.gov/apps/media/fact_sheets.asp.
3403	**Independent Payment Advisory Board (IPAB).** Creates an independent, 15-member Payment Advisory Board tasked with presenting Congress with comprehensive proposals to reduce excess cost growth and improve quality of care for Medicare beneficiaries. In years when Medicare costs are projected to exceed a target growth rate, the board's proposals will take effect unless Congress passes an alternative measure that achieves the same level of savings. Congress would be allowed to consider an alternative provision on a fast-track basis. Appropriates from the Medicare trust funds $15 million for FY2012 and, for each subsequent fiscal year, an amount equal to the previous fiscal year's appropriation adjusted for inflation.	Advisory reports may be submitted to Congress beginning Jan. 15, 2014.	The IPAB members have yet to be appointed by the President, with the advice and consent of the Senate.

ACA Section	Summary of Provision	Selected Deadlines	Implementation Actions Taken
PREVENTIVE AND PRIMARY CARE			
2602	**Coverage and Payment Coordination for Dual Eligibles.** Requires the Secretary, as part of the President's budget submission, to issue an annual report to Congress with recommendations for legislative action that would improve care coordination and benefits for dual-eligible individuals.	Annual report due each February with the President's budget.	Pursuant to ACA Sec. 2602, HHS established the Federal Coordinated Health Care Office (FCHC) and published a statement of its organization, functions, and delegations of authority on Dec. 30, 2010 (75 *Federal Register* 82405). See https://www.cms.gov/medicare-medicaid-coordination/. In fulfillment of the annual reporting requirement, HHS issued a letter to the Vice President and to Congress on Mar. 1, 2011 that reports on early FCHC activities. On Apr. 14, 2011, the FCHC announced the award of demonstration grants to 15 States. On May 16, 2011, the FCHC published a Request for Information (76 *Federal Register* 28196) on opportunities to better align benefits and incentives to prevent cost shifting and improve access to care for dual eligibles. On July 8, 2011, CMS issued guidance on financing models to support state efforts to integrate care for dual eligibles in a State Medicaid Director letter (SMDL #11-008 ACA #18).
2703	**Medicaid Health Home Option** Provides states with the option of enrolling Medicaid beneficiaries with chronic conditions in a health home. Requires the Secretary to establish standards for qualification as a designated provider of health home services.	States may elect option beginning Jan. 1, 2011	On Nov. 16, 2010, CMS issued preliminary guidance in a State Medicaid Director letter (SMDL #10-024, ACA #12). States had the option of electing the health home option since January 1, 2011. As of December 2011, Rhode Island and Missouri had approved State Plan Amendments with health home provisions.
3024	**Medicare Independence at Home Demonstration Program.** Requires the Secretary to conduct a three-year Medicare demonstration program to test a payment incentive and service delivery model aimed at reducing expenditures and improving health outcomes that uses physician- and nurse practitioner-directed primary care teams to provide home-based services to chronically ill patients. The Secretary must submit a plan, no later than Jan. 1, 2016, for expanding the program if it is determined that such expansion would improve the quality of care and reduce spending. Transfers $5 million from the Medicare trust funds for each of FY2010 through FY2015 for the demonstration (i.e., $30 million in total).	Demonstration to begin by Jan. 1, 2012.	In December 2011, CMS released a solicitation. Deadlines for the submission of applications and letters of intent vary depending on the application. The first deadline is February 6, 2012. For more information, including the application, visit: https://www.cms.gov/demoprojectsevalrpts/md/itemdetail.asp?itemid=CMS1240082 For a fact sheet on the independence at home demonstration, see http://www.cms.gov/DemoProjectsEvalRpts/downloads/IAH_FactSheet.pdf.
3026	**Community-Base Care Transitions Program** Requires the Secretary to establish a five-year program to provide funding to eligible hospitals and community-based organizations that provide evidence-based transition services to Medicare beneficiaries with multiple chronic conditions who are at high risk for hospital readmission. Transfers $500 million from the Medicare trust funds for the period FY2011 through FY2015.	Program to begin Jan. 1, 2011.	On Nov. 18, 2011, CMS announced the first seven sites to be selected for the CCTP. On March 14, 2012, CMS announced 23 additional participants in the program, and will continue to accept applications on a rolling basis until its funding is obligated. For a fact sheet on CCTP, see http://www.cms.gov/DemoProjectsEvalRpts/downloads/CCTP_FactSheet.pdf

ACA Section	Summary of Provision	Selected Deadlines	Implementation Actions Taken
3140	**Hospice Concurrent Care Demonstration Program.** Directs the Secretary to establish a three-year demonstration program, in up to 15 hospice programs in both rural and urban areas, that would allow patients who are eligible for hospice care also to receive all other Medicare covered services during the same period of time. Requires the Secretary to evaluate the impacts of the demonstration on patient care, quality of life, and spending in the Medicare program.	No specified deadlines.	This provision has not received the funding needed to commence implementation.
3502	**Community Health Team Grants to Support Medical Homes.** Requires the Secretary to award grants to or enter into contracts with eligible entities to support community-based interdisciplinary, inter-professional health teams in assisting primary care practices. Funding must be used to establish the health teams and to provide capitated payments to the providers. Authorizes the appropriation of SSAN for the program.	No specified deadlines.	This provision has not received the funding needed to commence implementation.
3503	**Medication Therapy Management (MTM) Grants.** Requires the Secretary to provide grants to support MTM services provided by licensed pharmacists that are targeted at patients who take four or more prescribed medications, take high-risk medications, have two or more chronic diseases, or have undergone a transition of care or other factors that are likely to create a high risk for medication-related problems. Authorizes the appropriation of SSAN for the program.	Grant program to begin by May 1, 2010.	This provision has not received the funding needed to commence implementation.
4001	**National Prevention, Health Promotion and Public Health Council.** Requires the President to establish an interagency National Prevention, Health Promotion and Public Health Council, chaired by the U.S. Surgeon General, tasked with developing a strategy across Federal departments to prevent disease and promote the nation's health.	National strategy due by Mar. 23, 2011.	The Council published the National Prevention Strategy on June 16, 2011, and the 2011 Annual Status Report on July 1, 2011. See http://www.healthcare.gov/center/councils/nphpphc/index.html.
4108	**Medicaid Prevention and Wellness Incentives.** Requires the Secretary to award state grants to provide incentives to Medicaid beneficiaries who successfully participate in evidence-based healthy lifestyle programs to prevent or help manage chronic disease. Appropriates $100 million for the five-year period Jan. 1, 2011, through Dec. 31, 2015.	Initial report due to Congress by Jan. 1, 2014.	The availability of funds for the Medicaid Incentives for Prevention of Chronic Diseases (MIPCD) program was announced in February 2011, with a May 2011 application deadline. See http://www.cms.gov/MIPCD/. On September 13, 2011, the following States were selected to receive grants: Wisconsin, Minnesota, New York, Nevada, New Hampshire, Montana, Hawaii, Texas, California, and Connecticut.

ACA Section	Summary of Provision	Selected Deadlines	Implementation Actions Taken
4201	**Community Transformation Grants (CTG).** Requires the Secretary to award grants for the implementation, evaluation, and dissemination of evidence-based community preventive health activities. Authorizes the appropriation of SSAN for each of FY2010 through FY2014 for the grant program.	Applications were due by July 2011.	In FY2011, approximately $103 million in prevention funding was awarded to a total of 61 states and communities. Twenty-six states and communities will use awarded grants to build capacity for community prevention efforts. Thirty-five states and communities will use awarded grants to implement evidence- and practice-based programs designed to improve health and wellness. See http://www.cdc.gov/communitytransformation/.
4202(a)	**Community Wellness Pilot Program.** Requires the Secretary to award grants for a five-year pilot program to provide community prevention interventions, screenings, and clinical referrals for individuals aged 55 to 64. Authorizes the appropriation of SSAN for each of FY2010 through FY2014 for the pilot program.	No specified deadlines.	This provision has not received the funding needed to commence implementation.
4202(b)	**Medicare Prevention and Wellness Evaluation.** Requires the Secretary to conduct an evaluation of community-based prevention and wellness programs and, based on the findings, develop a plan to promote healthy lifestyles and chronic disease self-management among Medicare beneficiaries. Requires the Secretary to transfer $50 million from the Medicare trust funds to fund the evaluation.	Report due to Congress by Sept. 30, 2013.	To date, no action has been taken on this provision.
5604	**Co-Locating Primary and Specialty Care in Community-Based Mental Health Settings.** Requires the Secretary to fund demonstration projects for providing coordinated and integrated services to individuals with mental illness and co-occurring chronic diseases through the co-location of primary and specialty care services in community-based mental and behavioral health settings. Authorizes the appropriation of $50 million for FY2010, and SSAN for each of FY2011 through FY2014 for the demonstration projects.	No specified deadlines.	This provision has not received the funding needed to commence implementation.
10333	**Community-Based Collaborative Care Network Program.** Authorizes the Secretary to award grants to eligible entities to support community-based collaborative care networks (CCNs). An eligible CCN is a consortium of health care providers with a joint governance structure that provides comprehensive coordinated and integrated health care services for low-income populations. CCNs must include a safety net hospital and all the federally-qualified health centers in the community. Authorizes the appropriation of SSAN for each of FY2011 through FY2015 for the CCN program.	No specified deadlines.	This provision has not received the funding needed to commence implementation.

ACA Section	Summary of Provision	Selected Deadlines	Implementation Actions Taken
QUALITY MEASUREMENT AND REPORTING			
2701	**Medicaid Adult Health Quality Measures.** Requires the Secretary to identify and publish for comment a recommended core set of adult health quality measures for use in State Medicaid programs. Appropriates $60 million for each of FY2010 through FY2014 (i.e., $300 million in total).	Notice of recommended measures due by Jan. 1, 2011.	On Dec. 30, 2010, the Secretary published a notice with comment period (75 *Federal Register* 82397) identifying an initial core set of health quality measures recommended for Medicaid eligible adults. The initial core set of measures may be viewed at: https://s3.amazonaws.com/public-inspection.federalregister.gov/2011-33756.pdf. The measures are also at: http://federalregister.gov/a/2011-33756. On December 30, 2011, the Secretary released the initial core set of quality measures.
3004	**Quality Measures Reporting System for Long-Term Care Facilities.** Requires long-term care hospitals, inpatient rehabilitation hospitals, and hospice programs to submit quality date starting in 2014. These facilities will face a two percent reduction in their annual update, increase factor for payment, or market basket (respectively) for failing to submit such data.	The Secretary must publish quality measures for the three facilities by October 1, 2012.	CMS published quality measures for all three facilities in the *Federal Register*: • On August 2, 2011, the rules specifying the quality measures to be reported by hospices and inpatient rehabilitation facilities were published. • On August 18, 2011, the rule for long-term care facilities was published as part of the final rule for "Hospital Inpatient Prospective Payment Systems for Acute Care Hospital" and "Long-Term Care Hospital Prospective Payment System and FY2012 Rates."
3005	**Quality Reporting for Cancer Hospitals.** Requires cancer hospitals to submit quality data starting in FY2014.	Quality measures selected for reporting must be published by 2014.	The Administration is working on a rule regarding quality measures for cancer hospitals, but it has not yet been published.
3011	**National Strategy for Health Care Quality.** Requires the Secretary to establish and submit to Congress a national strategy to improve the delivery of health care services, patient health outcomes, and population health. Requires the Secretary to create a website to make available information regarding (1) national priorities for health care quality improvement; (2) agency-specific strategic plans for health care quality; and (3) other information, as the Secretary determines to be appropriate.	National strategy due by Jan. 1, 2011.	On Mar. 21, 2011, HHS released "Report to Congress: National Strategy for Quality Improvement in Health Care." See http://www.healthcare.gov/center/reports/nationalqualitystrategy032011.pdf. AHRQ has created a webpage called "Working for Quality," which includes information about the National Quality Strategy. No information about the agency-specific strategic plans is posted. The National Quality Strategy states that development of these plans will require "additional collaboration and engagement of the participating agencies along with (the) private sector." See http://www.ahrq.gov/workingforquality/.
3012	**Interagency Working Group on Health Care Quality.** Requires the Interagency Working Group on Health Care Quality, convened by the President and chaired by the Secretary, to submit to Congress, and publish on the Internet, a report on its progress and recommendations.	Initial report due by Dec. 31, 2010; reports due annually thereafter.	The Interagency Working Group on Health Care Quality has been convened, consisting of 23 senior Federal officials. See http://www.ahrq.gov/workingforquality/. The first annual report was sent to Congress on March 21, 2011. HHS is developing the second annual report.

ACA Section	Summary of Provision	Selected Deadlines	Implementation Actions Taken
3013; 10303	**Quality Measure Development.** Requires the Secretary, in consultation with AHRQ and CMS to identify gaps in quality measures and award grants to eligible entities for the development of quality measures. Requires 10 provider-level outcome measures be developed for both acute and chronic disease and primary and preventive care.	Initial set of quality measures should be made public by March 23, 2012. The acute and chronic disease measures must be published by March 23, 2012, and the primary and prevent care measures by March 23, 2013.	HHS requested an expedited review by the National Quality Forum of readmissions measures. To date, HHS has not released provider-level outcomes measures for acute and chronic disease or primary or preventive care.
3014	**Quality Measurement.** Expands the duties of the consensus-based entity under contract with CMS pursuant to SSA Sec. 1890 (currently the National Quality Forum, NQF). Requires the entity to convene multi-stakeholder groups to provide input on the national priorities for health care quality improvement (developed under ACA) and on the selection of quality and efficiency measures for Medicare payment systems and other health care programs, and for reporting performance information to the public. Establishes a multi-step pre-rulemaking process and timeline for the adoption, dissemination, and review of measures by the Secretary.	In the pre-rulemaking process, the Secretary must make publicly available the initial list of measures under consideration by Dec. 1, 2011.	The NQF is serving as the convener of the multi-stakeholder groups defined in this section, and has established the Measure Applications Partnership (MAP) to carry out its convening duties. MAP, will provide pre-rulemaking input to HHS on the selection of measures for Federal payment and public reporting programs. As required by statute, a list of measures under consideration for 2012 rulemaking has been posted on NQF's website (see http://www.qualityforum.org/MAP/). On Feb. 1, 2012, MAP provided a report to HHS, based on this list of measures, recommending measures for inclusion in quality programs. In addition (although not required by statute), MAP has provided three reports as of Oct. 1, 2011; final reports for the clinician and safety coordination strategies, and an interim report for the dual-eligible beneficiaries quality measurement strategy (with a final report due June 1, 2012). Final reports for the dual-eligible beneficiaries quality measurement strategy and the remaining two workgroups (hospital and post-acute/long-term care) are expected by June 2012.
3015; 10305	**Data Collection; Public Reporting.** Requires the Secretary to collect and aggregate data on quality and resource use measure from information systems used to support health care delivery. A strategic framework for public reporting of performance information must be established.	No specified deadlines.	To date, no action has been taken on this provision.
6301	**Patient-Centered Outcomes Research.** Establishes a private, nonprofit entity—the Patient-Centered Outcomes Research Institute (PCORI)—governed by a public-private sector board appointed by the Comptroller General to identify priorities for and support comparative effectiveness research. Prohibits any research findings to be construed as mandates on practice guidelines or coverage decisions and contains patient safeguards to protect against discriminatory coverage decisions by HHS based on age, disability, terminal illness, or an individual's quality of life preference. Provides funding for PCORI over the 10-year period FY2010 through FY2019 through a mixture of annual appropriations and transfers from the Medicare trust funds.	Requires annual GAO reviews of PCORI's financial audits, research activities, etc. by Apr. 1.	GAO announced the appointments to the PCORI Board of Governors on Sept. 23, 2010. PCORI issued its first call for pilot projects in the fall of 2011. There were 856 grant applications submitted for the first call, of which a total of 40 pilots will be funded. PCORI also released a draft of its "National Priorities for Research" and "Research Agenda" for public comment. For more information, see http://www.pcori.org/.

ACA Section	Summary of Provision	Selected Deadlines	Implementation Actions Taken
10322	**Quality Reporting for Psychiatric Hospitals.** Requires psychiatric hospitals to submit quality data beginning in 2014. Failure to report this data will result in a two percentage point reduction in a facilities' annual update to their Federal rate for discharges.	Quality measures for psychiatric hospitals must be published by Oct. 1, 2012.	CMS intends to propose quality measures and reporting requirements through rule-making prior to Oct. 1, 2012. The agency is seeking input from the psychiatric community, and held two "listening sessions" with stakeholders in 2011 to discuss the measures they are considering.
ADMINISTRATION SIMPLIFICATION			
1104; 10109	**HIPAA Electronic Transactions Standards.** Establishes a timeline, with multiple deadlines through Jan. 1, 2016, for the Secretary to adopt and implement a single set of operating rules for each HIPAA administrative and financial electronic transaction for which there is an existing standard. Requires the Secretary to adopt a new electronic funds transfer standard and accompanying set of operating rules. Establishes penalty fees, beginning in 2014, for health plans that fail to certify that their data systems comply with the most current HIPAA standards and associated operating rules. As amended by 10109, the Secretary is required to solicit input on uniformity in financial and administrative activities from various stakeholders	Initial operating rules (health care claims status, health plan eligibility) due by July 1, 2011. Soliciting input on uniformity in financial and administrative activities by Jan. 1, 2012.	On July 8, 2011, HHS published an interim final rule adopting operating rules for health care claims status and health plan eligibility transactions (76 Federal Register 40458). The compliance date for the new operating rules is Jan. 1, 2013. For more information on ACA's administrative simplification provisions, see http://www.cms.gov/Affordable-Care-Act/. On January 5, 2012, HHS announced the Interim Final Regulation regarding new standards for electronic funds transfers. The regulation is effective January 1, 2012. All health plans covered under HIPAA must comply with the standards by January 1, 2014. This reform is estimated to save $4.5 billion off administrative costs from the adoption of electronic standards that will help eliminate inefficient manual processes. To view the IFR with comment period, see: http://ofr.gov/inspection.aspx.
1413	**Eligibility and Enrollment Systems.** Requires the Secretary to establish a system for the residents of each state to apply for enrollment in, receive a determination of eligibility for participation in, and continue participation in, applicable state health subsidy programs. The system must ensure that if any individual applying for an exchange is found to be eligible for Medicaid or the Children's Health Insurance Program (CHIP), then the individual is enrolled for assistance under that program.	No specified deadlines.	HHS released a final rule that implements the systems included in Section 1413 on March 12, 2012.
6105	**Standardized Complaint Form.** Requires the Secretary to develop and make available a standardized complaint form to be used by residents (or their representatives) in filing complaints against a skilled nursing facility (SNF) or a nursing facility	Effective Mar. 23, 2011.	CMS issued a letter to State Survey Agency Directors on March 18, 2011, announcing planned changes to the Nursing Home Compare Medicare website scheduled for Apr. 23, 2011, and July 21, 2011. The Apr. 23, 2011 changes will include a standardized complaint form and links to state complaint websites. See https://www.cms.gov/surveycertificationgeninfo/downloads/SCLetter11_17.pdf.

ACA Section	Summary of Provision	Selected Deadlines	Implementation Actions Taken
HEALTH INFORMATION TECHNOLOGY			
1561	**Enrollment Standards.** Requires the Secretary, in consultation with the Health Information Technology (HIT) Policy Committee and the HIT Standards Committee, to develop interoperable and secure standards and protocols that facilitate enrollment of individuals in federal and state health and human services programs.	Standards and protocols due by Sept. 19, 2010.	In Aug. 2010, the HIT Policy and Standards Committees approved initial recommendations for a minimum set of standards and data elements. On Sept. 17, 2010, the Secretary adopted these recommendations. See http://healthit.hhs.gov/portal/server.pt?open=512&mode=2&objID=3161.
6114	**Culture Change and Information Technology Demonstration Program.** Requires the Secretary, within one year of enactment (by Mar. 23, 2011), to award one or more competitive grants to support each of the following two three-year demonstration projects for SNFs and NFs: (1) develop best practices for culture change (i.e., patient-centric models of care); and (2) develop best practices for the use of health information technology. Authorizes the appropriation of SSAN for the demonstrations projects.	Award grants by March 23, 2011. Report due to Congress nine months after completion of the demo projects.	This provision has not received the funding needed to commence implementation.
10330	**CMS Computer System Modernization.** Requires the Secretary to develop and post on the department website a plan to modernize CMS's computer and data systems to support improvements in care delivery. The plan must include a detailed budget for the resources needed for its implementation.	Plan to be posted online by Dec. 23, 2010.	On Dec. 23, 2010, CMS released a report on its IT Modernization Program, "Modernizing CMS Computer and Data Systems to Support Improvements in Care Delivery, Version 1.0." See http://www4.cms.gov/InfoTechGenInfo/Downloads/CMSSection10330Plan.pdf.